Contents

Foreword

Nursing has for too long been the sleeping giant of our health services. Over the last decade, however, things have begun to change. Three years ago the first edition of *The Minor Illness Manual* captured this awakening as nurses began to take on the appraisal, diagnosis and treatment of minor illnesses within general practice. This second edition is launched upon a world in which the transformation of nurses into the major force for change within the NHS has been nothing short of dramatic.

Nurses provide 80% of direct patient care. Most people's experience of the health services begins and ends with a nurse and, increasingly, nurses now act as the patient's gateway to the NHS through schemes such as nurse-led general practices, NHS Direct and NHS walk-in centres. Nursing can at last be seen as a confident, forward-looking profession with enormous potential to prevent disease, provide high-quality care for the sick and promote healthy lifestyles.

Some things are slower to catch up, however. If nurses are to take on these new roles and new activities then how are they to be prepared? Where are the programmes of education that equip nurses with new skills and knowledge? How is this monitored and evaluated? And where is the equity that allows doctors and nurses, often doing the same job, to access the same high-quality continuing professional development? If change is to be sustained, and high-quality patient care placed at the centre of these changes, then more attention needs to be given to this issue by both employers and the Government alike.

The development of *Minor Illness: an open learning programme for nurse-led clinics in primary care,* by the authors of this manual, is a step in the right direction and is to be applauded. The next step should be learning aimed at doctors and nurses together. Professional evolution will slowly deconstruct the skills and knowledge hierarchy that defines our current boundaries.

This second edition of *The Minor Illness Manual* will provide a further valuable resource for nurses and doctors in general practice. Each copy deserves to quickly become dog-eared and well-thumbed. For our patients' sake, I hope this will be the case.

Pippa Gough
Director of Policy
Royal College of Nursing
June 2000

Foreword to the first edition

This is a book about the future shape of general practice in the United Kingdom.

Currently, throughout the country, patients are consulting nurses about their minor illnesses – be they coughs and colds, bumps and scrapes, tummy upsets, aches and pains, or worries and anxieties about this and that. The volume of this minor illness grows and grows as patients seek the unattainable goal of perfect health.

A carefully audited experiment in my own practice in suburban Stockton-on-Tees – a practice with a social class distribution about average for the United Kingdom – proved conclusively that patients like the opportunity to consult nurses about fairly trivial, but nevertheless bothersome minor symptoms, and acute short-term illness. Four out of every five patients did not need to be seen by a doctor and half simply needed advice and no prescription. This paper was published in the *British Medical Journal* after their customary rigorous review.[1] There were many, many requests for reprints from all types of general practice. Importantly there was no outcry from the medico-legal world. The system worked and the patients, once used to it, asked for nurse (not doctor) appointments on subsequent occasions.

But what was lacking in our experiment was a manual containing guidelines to help the nurse appraise, diagnose and treat the broad spectrum of minor illnesses that presented. Here is such a manual. It has been written by three busy general practitioners, in discussion with their practice nurses. What they have set down is the product of much thoughtful appraisal of their expertise in managing minor illnesses over many years.

For practices deciding to embark on this system of minor illness care, there are a few 'musts'. First, the nurses must be fully registered, experienced and preferably have undertaken a practice nurse training programme. Second, they must have a doctor immediately available to them whilst they are consulting; a quick word on the telephone will usually suffice, except for a few problems where the doctor will need to see the patient. Third, the reception and office staff must know the sort of problems that the nurse is happy to see when they make the appointments, and they must always provide a doctor appointment if they sense that this is the patient's preference.

Obviously not all minor illness will go to nurses; there is more than enough of it to go round! But with even a small proportion of it being seen by nurses, particularly the 'urgent', 'same-day' problems, it will release doctor time for the care and management of more complicated and serious conditions (which will increasingly devolve on to primary healthcare teams, as hospital empires contract).

I commend this book to all practice nurses and their GPs – it is a vital aid to finding a solution to the 'volume problem' of primary care in the United Kingdom.

Geoffrey Marsh MBE
February 1997

1   Marsh GN and Dawes ML (1995) Establishing a minor illness nurse in a busy general practice. *BMJ.* **310**: 778–80.

Preface

When the first edition of *The Minor Illness Manual* was published in 1997, the concept of a nurse-run minor illness clinic in primary care was new and controversial. Geoffrey Marsh's pioneering paper[1] had opened the door to a revolution in the provision of care to patients requesting 'same-day' appointments in general practice, but many doctors were doubtful about the ability of nurses to work in the front line where patients presented with vague, undifferentiated problems.

Three years on the situation is very different. A substantial amount of published research[2-5] has shown that nurses can do this work safely and efficiently, without compromising patient satisfaction. Changes to the structure of primary care have enabled nurse-led practices to be developed,[6] and the promotion of walk-in clinics by the Department of Health has increased public confidence in the nurse's role as the first point of contact for primary care.

How do nurses obtain relevant training for this role? Originally this was individual and practice-based. We have now developed an open learning pack, *Minor Illness: an open learning programme for nurse-led clinics in primary care*, which evolved from a university-accredited course of seminars and one-to-one teaching designed from our own practice. This new edition of the manual is intended for use as a desk-top *aide-mèmoire*. It is not a substitute for adequate training, and ideally should be used in conjunction with both a distance learning or taught course and a practical programme based in primary care. Such a course would provide insight into the reasons behind the management decisions in the manual, as well as an essential background in communication, pharmacology, microbiology and evidence-based practice.

Historically, the independent contractor status of the general practitioner has encouraged individualism. Those who work in large practices will find that there may be almost as many ways of managing a specific clinical problem as there are clinicians within the practice. This poses a difficulty in developing the guidelines which the nurse should follow.

Where possible we have quoted a systematic review of the literature to support our recommendations. Many of these are drawn from the Cochrane Library, an electronic compendium of 3000 reviews and over 200 000 clinical trials, which is updated quarterly. This should be available in your local hospital library, or your practice can subscribe to it on CD-Rom or via the Internet. Primary care groups may consider buying licences on behalf of their practices. Phone 020 7383 6185/6245 for more information.

Our suggestions in the first edition had to be cautious, until the role of the nurse in diagnosis and management had become less controversial and more firmly established. Three factors have encouraged us to be more radical in this edition:

- the national drive to reduce antibiotic prescribing[7]

- a growing body of evidence that antibiotics are often prescribed inappropriately[8]

- increasing confidence in the ability of nurses to manage urgent problems in primary care.

We hope that *The Minor Illness Manual* will continue to support decision making by specialist nurses. Such nurses are increasingly becoming the first point of contact for patients requesting same-day appointments in primary care.

Gina Johnson
Ian Hill-Smith
Chris Ellis
June 2000

1   Marsh G and Dawes N (1995) Establishing a minor illness nurse in a busy general practice. *BMJ*. **310**: 778–80.
2   Chambers N (1988) *Nurse Practitioners in Primary Care*. Radcliffe Medical Press, Oxford.
3   Myes P, Lenci B and Sheldon M (1997) A nurse practitioner as first point of contact for urgent medical problems in a general practice setting. *Family Practice*. **14**(6): 492–7.
4   Shum C, Humphreys A, Wheeler D *et al*. (2000) Nurse management of patients with minor illnesses in general practice: multicentre, randomised controlled trial. *BMJ*. **320**: 1038–43.
5   Kinnersley P, Anderson E, Parry K *et al*. (2000) Randomised controlled trial of nurse practitioner versus general practitioner care for patients requesting 'same day' consultations in primary care. *BMJ*. **320**: 1043–8.
6   Sibbald B (1996) Skill mix and professional roles in primary care. In: *What is the Future for a Primary-care Led NHS?* National Primary Care Research and Development Series. Radcliffe Medical Press, Oxford.
7   Department of Health Standing Medical Committee Sub-Group on Antimicrobial Resistance (1988) *The Path of Least Resistance*. Department of Health, London.
8   Butler C, Rollnick S, Kinnersley P *et al*. (1988) Reducing antibiotics for respiratory tract symptoms in primary care: consolidating 'why' and considering 'how'. *Br J Gen Pract*. **48**: 1865–70.

Preface to the first edition

Today primary care has to meet new demands: increasing patient expectations and the transfer of work previously done in hospital. Many practices have addressed this problem by extending the role of the practice nurse to include the management of minor illness, especially the 'extras' or 'emergencies' who request same-day appointments.

When our practice nurse started to develop her skills in this way, we could find no suitable book of guidelines; so we wrote one. The advice given is research-based wherever possible, but for many minor illnesses a consensus view must suffice.

This manual will enable an experienced practice nurse to manage most patients with minor illness, provided that she/he can also:

- educate patients in self-care

- examine the ears and throat, listen to the chest and feel the abdomen for tenderness

- take swabs for culture

- find information in the *British National Formulary* (BNF)

- appreciate that the patient may have hidden worries

- recognise when to seek help.

Experience shows that a nurse-run 'emergency clinic' is safe, liked by patients and encourages self-care. It frees the doctor to deal with more complex medical problems and reduces the need for locum cover. Such a scheme could also be adopted by student health services, accident and emergency departments and deputizing or cooperative services.

We have found the term 'emergency clinic' preferable to 'minor illness clinic'; patients object to the implication that their problems are minor.

Concern has been expressed about the legality and accountability of such a nurse-run clinic. The legal position was summarised by Sue Parker of the Medical Defence Union as follows:

> If a nurse works in a situation where she administers and/or supplies other types of therapy such as oral antibiotics without the patient being seen by the doctor, then the prescription should be signed by the doctor before the medicine is administered or dispensed.

The law does not prohibit a nurse making a diagnosis and deciding upon treatment but it does not allow the supply of a prescription-only medicine without a prescription. In order to satisfy the legal requirements the nurse should:

- decide what treatment is needed

- fill in the prescription as per the protocol

- obtain the appropriate practitioner's signature.

Any other sequence is unacceptable.

(*Community Nurse*, April 1996, 19–20)

We are most grateful to Dr Geoffrey Marsh, who pioneered the concept of the minor illness nurse and whose help and encouragement has been invaluable in the development of this book. We would like to thank Bedfordshire Health, who provided initial funding for the pilot scheme in our practice and who are encouraging its dissemination throughout the county. Many thanks also go to the staff of Stopsley Group Practice for their constant support.

Gina Johnson
Ian Hill-Smith
Chris Ellis
February 1997

Acknowledgements

We would like to thank our staff at the Stopsley Group Practice for their ongoing support, especially Lorraine Dakin, without whose skills and patience the Minor Illness Course would never have been possible. We are grateful to the many nurses who have attended our courses and seminars, who have taught us so much.

David Johnson, Medical Librarian at the Luton and Dunstable Hospital, provided invaluable help with researching the evidence.

We also thank our patients, for allowing us to learn from their experiences of minor illness.

The nurse's perspective: accessing appropriate support in order to achieve safe and effective practice

The development of a specialist role in the treatment of minor illnesses represents yet another advance in nursing practice. The Royal College of Nursing has defined nurse specialists as:

> experts in a particular aspect of nursing care … They demonstrate refined clinical practice, either as a result of significant experience or advanced expertise, or knowledge in a branch or speciality.[1]

Breaking the boundaries of previously defined roles and taking on new challenges are not, then, unfamiliar in nursing. Many practice nurses have already taken on expanded roles as specialist nurses in family planning or asthma, where diagnostic decisions are made and treatments recommended. The UKCC's *Scope of Professional Practice*[2] gives nurses, particularly those in primary care, more freedom to take on new roles by basing nursing on the patients' needs. Nevertheless, anxieties remain inherent in any new role and can subsequently affect the levels of stress experienced by nurses who take on the management of minor illness. It is essential that the processes at national, intermediate and individual levels are in place and accessible in order to promote both safe and effective practice. They are also needed to provide the necessary support to prevent undue stress and anxiety for the nurses practising in this specialist area.

The UKCC's *Code of Professional Conduct*[3] states that registered nurses are personally accountable for their practice and must:

- act always in such a manner as to promote and safeguard the interests and wellbeing of patients and clients
- ensure that no action or omission on [their] part, or within [their] sphere of responsibility, is detrimental to the interests, condition or safety of patients or clients
- maintain and improve [their] professional knowledge and competence
- acknowledge any limitations in [their] knowledge and competence and decline any duties and responsibilities unless able to perform them in a safe and skilled manner.

All nurses are familiar with the concept of professional and legal accountability. Some concerns have been expressed about the legality and accountability of nurse-led clinics for the management of minor illness. Sue Parker of the Nursing and Non-Medical Advisory Service of the Medical Defence

Union, was asked for her comments on the publication of the first edition of *The Minor Illness Manual* in 1997. She wrote:

> There is no legal reason why nurses should not run their own clinics, but this would be seen as a delegated task and both the doctor and the nurse are professionally accountable and may be legally liable. But if their practice can be supported by a substantial body of nursing and medical opinion, then it is likely that the patient will receive safe and therapeutic care and that both the doctor and nurse will protect their professional position.

Appropriate professional indemnity insurance is essential. In addition to the indemnity provided by the Royal College of Nursing, the Medical Defence Union and the Medical Protection Society have group schemes to cover both the general practitioners and the practice nurses within a practice. It is advisable to provide these bodies with copies of job descriptions for any minor illness specialist nurse working in practice.

At the intermediate or local level, employers are vicariously liable for the nurses they employ whether they are partnerships of doctors or NHS trusts. This covers liability for errors and omissions on the part of the nurse and an obligation to ensure that the nurses are suitably trained for the work that they undertake. However, it is also an obligation of all health professionals to refer patients with problems that are beyond their professional competence. Once a nurse has undertaken the appropriate education and assessment, protocols should be agreed so that newly acquired skills and competencies can be used appropriately. The Crown Review defines such protocols as 'general guidelines written or agreed by doctors under which specified medicines are administered or supplied by other health care professionals to patients in defined clinical circumstances'.[4] Protocols add legal security to the nurses' role and position.[5] Protocols should also conform to national criteria. The Royal College of Nursing has set out guidelines on the correct development, content and implementation of group protocols.[6] The College advises that protocols should include:

- the clinical problem and circumstances to which the protocol applies
- the delegating doctor, the name(s) of nurses, their education and qualifications
- a description of the treatments included under the protocol.

Group protocols should be agreed which reflect the level of confidence and ability of the specialist nurse in managing specific conditions. The guidelines in *The Minor Illness Manual* should be discussed so that they can be agreed and adapted to local needs. Where opinions differ as to the appropriate course of action or treatment, evidence of best practice should be the deciding factor. It is also important to have a job description so that the specialist nurse, the doctors and all the practice staff are aware of the new role and its boundaries.

Appropriate support at local level may also be accessed through clinical supervision, the benefits of which are widely documented. Its aims include offering support, facilitating professional autonomy and improving clinical practice. The NHS Executive takes its explanation of clinical supervision from *A Vision for the Future* (1993)[7] as:

> ... a formal process of professional support and learning which enables individual practitioners to develop knowledge and competence, assume responsibility for their own practice and enhance consumer protection and safety of care in complex clinical situations. It is central to the process of learning and to the expansion of the scope of practice and should be seen as a means of encouraging self-assessment and analytical and reflective skills.

Systems of clinical supervision are currently in place or being implemented at local levels and should be accessible to all nurses, whether GP- or trust-employed. Reflection is not exclusive to clinical supervision: it should also remain an integral part of practice at the individual level.[8] Reflection involves critical thinking and the interpretation of experiences in clinical practice, resulting in a changed perspective or knowledge. It is a valuable method of learning no matter how great a practitioner's experience. Moreover, learning through the process of reflection places control with the individual practitioner.

The establishment of nurse-led minor illness clinics has proved to be of enormous benefit. Patients appreciate the improved service, doctors find that they can work more effectively on specifically medical problems and receptionists feel less stressed because they have more options to offer patients who request same-day appointments. From the nurses' perspective, taking on this specialist role is rewarding because it has provided patients with safe, effective care and improved access to the Health Service. Providing education in the management of minor illness by specialist nurses has also increased the development of a culture of learning within the practice. The characteristics of this have been cited by the ENB as 'a willingness to experiment and try out new things, by support for reflective practice, and by the willingness to gain insight from experiments and experiences'.[9] Many rewards are being reaped, by both the practice team and the population it serves, through the development of this specialist nurse role in primary care.

1   Royal College of Nursing (1988) *Specialties in Nursing: a report of the working party investigating the development of specialties within the nursing profession.* RCN, London, p 6.
2   United Kingdom Central Council (1992) *Scope of Professional Practice.* UKCC, London.
3   United Kingdom Central Council (1992) *Code of Professional Conduct.* UKCC, London.
4   Crown Review Consultative Document HSC 97/47.
5   Medicines Act 58.2(b).
6   Royal College of Nursing (1988) *The supply and administration of medicines under group protocol arrangements.* Fact sheet No. 000922. RCN, London.
7   NHS Executive (1996) *Clinical Supervision: a resource pack for practice nurses.* Cited in the introductory Professional Letter 94/5 from the Chief Nursing Officer.
8   For an overview see Atkins S and Murphy K (1993) Reflection: a review of the literature. *J Adv Nurs.* **18**: 1188–92
9   English National Board for Nursing, Midwifery and Health Visiting (1994) *Lifelong Learners – partnerships for care,* p 11 citing Argyris and Schon (1978) ENB, London.

Introduction

General advice

History
- listening is the greatest skill
- open questions may reveal hidden concerns
- most diagnoses are made on the history – 'listen to the patient: he is telling you the diagnosis'

Examination
- this may reveal important signs, but will also serve to reassure the patient

Tests
- only useful if the management depends on the result

Action
- discuss the options and agree the proposed plan of management with the patient
- ask the patient to contact the practice again if:
  - the situation worsens
  - there is no improvement within a specified time

Caution
- we recognise that although guidelines support clinical judgement, they can never replace experience and intuition

Upper respiratory tract

Sore throat

History
- duration
- fever/malaise
- recurrent problems
- altered immunity (e.g. diabetes, leukaemia, acquired immunodeficiency syndrome (AIDS), taking cortico-steroids or carbimazole)

Examination
- examine throat
- tongue protrusion may reveal tonsils:
  - are they inflamed?
  - any white spots?
- use tongue depressor if back of throat not visible (but beware of epiglottitis, *see* below)
- check neck for enlarged lymph nodes (lymphadenopathy)
- macular rash (small red patches, not raised)

Test
- full blood count (FBC) and Paul Bunnell may be helpful to diagnose glandular fever, if symptoms persist for longer than a week

Action
- antibiotics are of no benefit if the infection is viral, and only shorten the duration of fever by 24 h if it is bacterial
- if less than three of the four Centor criteria (Box 1.1) are fulfilled, the infection is unlikely to be bacterial and antibiotics should not be considered

> **Box 1.1** Centor criteria (factors associated with an increased chance of bacterial infection)
>
> - History of fever
> - Absence of cough
> - Swollen tender anterior cervical lymph nodes
> - Tonsillar exudate

- in a teenager these symptoms and signs are more likely to be due to glandular fever, so antibiotics should generally be avoided unless there is severe malaise. Do not use amoxicillin, which may cause a rash in a patient with glandular fever (this is disease-specific, not due to an allergy). Consider tests above

- a macular rash on the trunk may be due to a generalised streptococcal infection (scarlatina) – *see* page 38

Prescription/OTC
- symptomatic treatment for most patients (ibuprofen or paracetamol)

- if an antibiotic is indicated:

  - in adults and children 10 and over, penicillin V tablets or suspension for 7 days (10 days if recurrent problems)

  - in children under 10, amoxicillin suspension (tastes better than penicillin V) for 7–10 days

  - if allergic to penicillin, use erythromycin

Refer to GP
- immediately if:

  - child very sick, drooling, cannot swallow (possible *epiglottitis*, do not examine throat)

  - large swelling around one tonsil (possible *quinsy*, may need surgery)

Both of these are very rare.

  - altered immunity

- Del Mar C and Glasziou P (1988) Antibiotics for the symptoms and complications of sore throat (Cochrane Review). In: *Cochrane Library*, Issue 2. Update Software, Oxford, updated quarterly.
- Little P, Williamson I, Warner G *et al.* (1997) Open randomised trial of prescribing strategies in managing sore throat. *BMJ.* **314**: 722–7.
- Zwart S, Sachs A, Gijs J *et al.* (2000) Penicillin for acute sore throat: randomised double blind trial of seven days versus three days treatment or placebo in adults. *BMJ.* **320**: 150–4.
- Centor RM, Witherspoon JM, Dalton HP *et al.* (1981) The diagnosis of strep throat in adults in the emergency room. *Med Decis Making.* **1**: 239–46.

'Swollen glands' (enlarged cervical lymph nodes)

History	• sore throat?
	• duration of swelling
Examination	• number and size of enlarged nodes
	• throat
Test	• FBC and Paul Bunnell if symptoms last more than a week in a teenager or young adult
Action	• explain that the 'glands' are the body's defence against infection
Prescription/OTC	• ibuprofen or paracetamol if pain is severe
Refer to GP	• if there is a single very large painful node (may contain an abscess)
	• if lymph nodes are enlarging progressively (may be a sign of lymphoma, leukaemia or tuberculosis)

Earache

History	• duration of pain
	• fever
	• deafness
	• discharge
	• recent swimming
	• previous attacks (how treated and what happened)

Examination
- look at canal:
    - inflammation
    - discharge
    - swelling (general or local, e.g. boil)
- look at eardrum:
    - colour
    - perforation
    - bulging/retracted
    - fluid level

Tests
- take ear swab (being careful not to puncture the drum) if:
    - recent history of swimming
    - not responding to initial treatment
    - or copious discharge

Action
- depends on diagnosis – *see* subsections:
    - otitis media
    - otitis externa
    - boil in ear canal
    - eustachian catarrh

Otitis media

Otitis media causes pain, deafness and sometimes fever, vomiting and loss of balance. The eardrum is red. It may be bulging or a discharge may be present. If the history is suggestive but the drum cannot be seen (e.g. because of wax) it is safest to assume that otitis media is present. Pink eardrums are to be expected if other membranes are inflamed (e.g. conjunctivitis, red throat), or after crying. Antibiotics are not necessary for these patients.

Action
- recommend regular analgesia
- give antibiotics to children under 2 years old
- explain that antibiotics are not helpful for the majority of patients with otitis media. 60% of patients will be pain-free within 24 h

- the chances of experiencing a side effect from the antibiotic are greater than the chances of benefiting

- if patient/parent is unhappy with this advice, consider offering an antibiotic prescription for use if there is no improvement within 48 h

- reassure that ear infections very rarely cause permanent hearing damage

- patients with otitis media should not fly

- severe infections may cause temporary deafness by perforation of the eardrum, which will usually heal in a few weeks

Prescription/OTC • paracetamol or ibuprofen

- if antibiotic indicated:

  – amoxicillin for 5 days

  – erythromycin if the patient is allergic to penicillin

  – if not responding to the above treatment change to co-amoxiclav (trimethoprim if allergic to penicillin)

Refer to GP • make appointment

  – if hearing does not return to normal within 14 days

  – if more than six episodes of otitis media per year

- Glasziou P, Hayem M and Del Mar C (1998) *Antibiotic versus placebo for acute otitis media in children* (Cochrane Review). In: *Cochrane Library*, Issue 2. Update Software, Oxford, updated quarterly.

Otitis externa

This causes itchy discomfort rather than pain. Insertion of the auriscope is often uncomfortable. The canal looks irregular, red or moist, perhaps with discharge.

Test • take swab if there is copious discharge

Action • recommend cotton wool and Vaseline to keep water out of inflamed ears while showering or washing hair

- recommend avoidance of swimming while ear is inflamed

- advise patient that swimming may cause a recurrence

Prescription
- give Otosporin eardrops for 7 days

Refer to GP
- if persistent/recurrent symptoms, for consideration of ear, nose and throat (ENT) referral

- Halpern H, Palmer C and Seidlin M (1999) Treatment patterns for otitis externa. *JABFP.* **12**(1): 1–7.

Boil in ear canal

This causes a localised red swelling in the canal, often with severe pain on insertion of the auriscope.

Action
- give oral flucloxacillin for 5 days, or erythromycin if the patient is allergic to penicillin
- warn the patient that the ear may discharge

Eustachian catarrh

The hearing is impaired and the ear is intermittently uncomfortable. The eardrum may appear normal, retracted or bulging. A fluid level may be seen behind the drum, which is not inflamed.

Action
- explain that the eardrum is a sensitive structure that hurts when the pressure changes. When catarrh blocks the eustachian tube, changes in atmospheric pressure cause earache that comes and goes
- try to 'pop' the ears

Prescription/OTC
- paracetamol for children
- steam inhalations for adults
- pseudoephedrine may give temporary relief, but *see* the contraindications and cautions in the Formulary

Colds and 'flu

Be aware that although most patients with a 'flu-like illness will indeed have a simple viral infection, there are many rare diseases that give the same initial symptoms. If the history has some odd features, or if the symptoms have been going on rather too long for a simple cold, then ask open general questions to see if there could be an alternative source of infection (such as the urinary tract).

History	• duration
	• fever
	• foreign travel
	• joint and muscle pains
	• sinus pain
	• earache
	• productive cough
	• urinary symptoms
	• what medicine tried?

Examination
- ears
- throat
- chest
- tenderness over sinuses

} if there are relevant symptoms

Tests
- none

Action
- if sinusitis / otitis media / cough with crackles in chest, refer to relevant section
- if not, explain the nature of viral infections and stress that antibiotics will not help (anaphylactic reactions to penicillin are ten times more common than serious adverse reactions to DTP (diphtheria, tetanus, pertussis) vaccination)

Prescription/OTC
- paracetamol or ibuprofen
- steam inhalations
- saline nose drops for babies
- chlorpheniramine at night for congestion
- pseudoephedrine (*see* cautions in Formulary)
- zinc lozenges (Strepsils Zinc Defence™) bought over the counter for about £3 shorten the duration of colds

Refer to GP	• if the symptoms do not fit comfortably with a diagnosis of a cold or 'flu
	• if recent travel to malarious/tropical region
Caution	• do not confuse with hayfever (no fever, recurrent spring symptoms)
	• if high fever, *see* cautions in fever section, page 18

• Mossad S, Macknin M and Medendorp S (1996) Zinc gluconate lozenges for treating the common cold. A randomized, double-blind, placebo-controlled study. *Ann Intern Med.* **125**: 81–8. (Also in *Evidence Based Medicine* 1996; **1**(7): 204.)

Sinusitis

History	• duration
	• fever
	• facial pain worse on bending head forwards
	• purulent nasal or post-nasal discharge
	• previous episodes: how treated?
Examination	• tenderness over sinuses
	• throat
	• ears
Tests	• none
Action	• stop smoking
Prescription/OTC	• analgesia with paracetamol or ibuprofen
	• steam inhalations with menthol and eucalyptus
	• antibiotics are of marginal benefit. Consider amoxicillin for 7 days (or erythromycin if the patient is allergic to penicillin)
Refer to GP	• same day if:
	– severe illness
	– swelling around the eyes or on forehead

Refer to dentist • if unilateral maxillary sinusitis (may be secondary to dental infection)

• Lindbaek M, Hjortdahl P and Johnsen U (1996) Randomised double blind placebo controlled trial of penicillin V and amoxycillin in the treatment of acute sinus infections in adults. *BMJ*. **313**: 325–9.
• Little D, Mann B and Sherk D (1998) Factors influencing the clinical diagnosis of sinusitis. *J Fam Prac*. **46**(2): 147–52.

Cough

History
- duration
- dry/productive/wheezy
- colour of sputum
- fever
- chest pain
- breathlessness
- previous similar episodes (how treated and what happened?)
- known chest problems
- smoking (amount, duration)

Examination
- pallor/cyanosis
- confusion
- fever
- respiratory rate
- crackles in chest (where located?)
- wheezing
- subcostal/intercostal recession in babies
- ears and throat in children (otitis media and tonsillitis may coexist)

Tests
- peak flow rate if asthma suspected in adult or child over 5 years (*see* section on acute asthma, page 13)

Action
- stress '*antibiotics do not cure virus infections*'
- adequate fluid intake
- steam inhalations two to three times a day
- stop smoking (includes parents of coughing child)
- give antibiotics if:
  - sputum brown or bloodstained
  - severe malaise
  - crackles in the chest
  - history of chronic obstructive pulmonary disease (COPD)/bronchiectasis
  - smoker over 55

Prescription/OTC
- if antibiotics indicated, give amoxicillin for 5 days (or erythromycin if allergic to penicillin)
- if not responding to amoxicillin and further antibiotics indicated, add doxycycline or change to erythromycin
- pholcodine linctus may be helpful (though not curative) to soothe an irritating cough
- pseudoephedrine may be helpful if there is marked nasal congestion (*see* cautions in Formulary)
- if wheezing in child under 5 years either:
  - salbutamol via Volumatic (can be used with paediatric mask for children of 2 years or younger) 100 µg single dose four times a day
- **or** if unable to use Volumatic:
  - terbutaline syrup
- if wheezing in older child or adult:
  - bronchodilator, inhaled salbutamol or equivalent, appropriate to age and capability, four times a day for up to 1 week
  - if not better or still needing bronchodilator after 1 week, recommend review appointment with doctor

Refer to GP
- urgently if:
  - baby with rapid respirations, intercostal/subcostal recession, wheezes or crackles (may be bronchiolitis)
  - cyanosis

– mental confusion

– very unwell or distressed

– peak flow rate below 75% of predicted value

– one-sided chest pain, worse on coughing or deep breathing (suggests pleurisy, pneumonia, pulmonary embolism or pneumothorax)

- make appointment if persistent or recurrent symptoms

Caution
- danger signs are moderate to severe breathlessness, distress, chest pain, cyanosis, pallor, subcostal/intercostal recession and raised respiratory rate in children

- beware of asthmatics who look ill, but have passed from the wheezy to the non-wheezy phase. Experienced asthmatics will tell you how bad they are and usually know what is needed from previous episodes

- Fahey T, Stocks N and Thomas T (1998) Quantitative systematic review of randomised controlled trials comparing antibiotic with placebo for acute cough in adults. *BMJ.* **316**: 906–10.

Box 1.2 Notes on cough

Cough is a very common presenting symptom. Beware that some patients call any episode of coughing 'bronchitis', whatever its true cause. Other symptoms may accompany it and help to make a diagnosis. The patient may present because the cough is persistent or interferes with sleep, or because of anxiety that infection is 'going to the chest'. Quite often a friend or relative has suggested that the patient should seek medical help.[1] Mothers may fear that their children will choke in the night.[2]

Cough may be due to:

(a) infection. This is the *commonest* cause of a cough in general practice. Most are viral but some are caused by primary or secondary infection with bacteria;

(b) physical and chemical stimuli, e.g. cold air, cigarette smoke;

(c) circulatory problems. A persistent dry cough in the elderly, with crackles at the lung bases, is likely to be due to heart failure. Dry coughs following sudden chest pain may be due to pulmonary embolism;

continued overleaf

(d) cancer. A persistent cough in a smoker, associated with chest pain or weight loss, is suspicious;

(e) iatrogenic. Cough is commonly caused by angiotensin-converting enzyme inhibitors (drug names ending in '-april');

(f) habit.

A persistent or relapsing cough may occur in:

- asthmatics (young children may present with cough without wheezing)
- heavy smokers (but beware cancer)
- small children with catarrh
- whooping cough (rare, thanks to immunisation)
- *Mycoplasma pneumoniae*, an unusual type of infection which occurs in cycles of 3–5 years. It causes a cough which may last for 3 months. It is sensitive to erythromycin or doxycycline, but not amoxicillin. A 2-week course is necessary
- tuberculosis.

After a viral infection the cough may last for some weeks. Patients somehow expect proprietary cough medicines to cure the cough and come for something stronger because brand X 'hasn't worked'. They need gentle re-education. Pholcodine linctus may be helpful (although not curative) to soothe an irritating cough.

1　Zola IK (1973) Pathways to the doctor: from person to patient. *Soc Sci Med.* **7**: 677–89.
2　Cornford CS, Morgan M and Ridsdale L (1993) Why do mothers consult when their children cough? *Fam Pract.* **10**: 193–6.

Croup

A viral infection of children aged between 3 months and 5 years.

History	• cough (often 'brassy' or 'barking')
	• crowing noise on inspiration (stridor, worse at night)
Examination	• breathless?
	• respiratory rate
	• listen to chest (usually normal)
	• examine throat

Action	• explain nature of illness
	• steam inhalations are often used but their effectiveness is not proven
Refer to GP	• immediately for consideration of single dose of oral steroid

• Ausejo M, Saenz A, Pham B *et al*. (1999) The effectiveness of glucocorticoids in treating croup: meta-analysis. *BMJ*. **319**: 595–600.
• Cates C (1999) Suitable formulations of oral glucocorticoids are available in primary care. *BMJ*. **319**: 1577.

Acute asthma

Nurses vary in their confidence in dealing with asthma. Asthma-trained nurses will be able to manage more severe cases.

History	• known asthmatic?
	• previous admission to hospital?
	• duration of symptoms:
	– wheeze
	– breathlessness
	– cough, especially at night
	– tightness in the chest
	• personal/family history of atopy – hayfever, eczema
	• present and previous medication
	• smoker (if a child, do parents or carers smoke?)
	• fever
	• chest pain
Examination	• ability to complete sentences
	• pallor/cyanosis
	• respiratory rate
	• pulse rate
	• subcostal/intercostal recession

- listen to chest for wheezes/crackles (crackles suggest an infection; *see* cough, page 9)

Tests
- peak flow rate (PFR)

- compare with predicted rate from charts (*see* Figures 1.1 and 1.2), and the patient's usual rate

Action
Adults and children over 5 years with PFR greater than 75% of expected value

- give usual inhaled bronchodilator. Check PFR afterwards

- check inhaler technique

- commence inhaled beclometasone, or double the dose of existing inhaled corticosteroid

- consider prescribing peak flow meter if patient does not already have one

- recommend recording the results on a chart

- advise the patient to seek further medical help if the asthma worsens despite the increase in treatment

- follow-up in 1–2 weeks for review of long-term treatment

Children 5 years and younger with mild symptoms

- try usual bronchodilator or, if uncooperative, nebulised salbutamol 2.5 mg

- observe, assess effect, listen to the chest again

- consider regular preventative therapy, or double dose of existing therapy

- continue inhaled bronchodilator, but ensure adequate technique

- if inadequate, consider changing the inhaler delivery system, e.g. to a volumatic, breath-actuated device, or provide short-term loan of nebuliser and prescription for nebules

- advise parents to seek further medical help if the asthma worsens: child more distressed, breathing faster, wheezing more, recession

- review after 1–7 days depending on severity and parental confidence in dealing with asthma

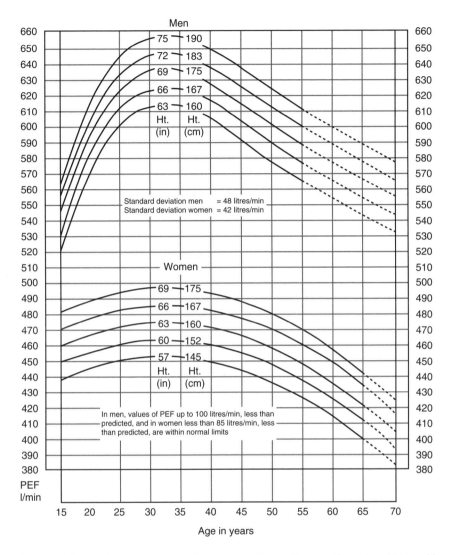

Figure 1.1 Peak expiratory flow in normal subjects. (Source: Gregg I and Nunn AJ (1973) Peak expiratory flow in normal subjects. *BMJ*. **3**: 282–4.)

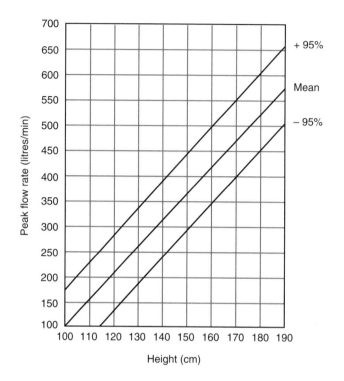

This nomogram results from tests carried out by Dr S Godfrey and his colleagues on a sample of 382 normal boys and girls aged 5–18 years. Each child blew five times into a standard Wright peak flow meter and the highest reading was accepted in each case. All measurements were completed within a 6-week period. The outer lines of the graph indicated that the results of 95% of children fell within these boundaries.

Figure 1.2   Peak expiratory flow in children. (Source: Godfrey S et al. (1970) Spirometry, lung volumes and airway resistance in normal children aged 5 to 18 years. Br J Dis Chest. **64**: 15–24.)

Refer to GP • immediately if:
  – silent chest
  – cyanosis
  – exhaustion
  – slow pulse
  – PFR below 75% of predicted rate
  – child: distressed; respiratory rate over 40/minute; recession; widespread wheezes

– chest pain (suggests asthma is complicated by pleurisy, pneumothorax or pulmonary embolus)

Fever

History
- duration
- degree (if accurate thermometer used)
- any other symptoms?
- sore throat/cold
- cough
- dysuria/frequency
- vomiting/diarrhoea
- rash
- travel to tropical area in last 3 months

Examination (as suggested by symptoms)
- ears
- throat
- cervical lymph nodes
- chest
- spots (beware the petechial rash of meningitis)
- photophobia
- neck stiffness (e.g. can a child kiss his knees?)
- lethargy, drowsiness
- breasts in lactating women
- any painful area (e.g. sinuses, abdomen)

Tests
- test urine for protein and blood nitrites if cause of fever not obvious (to avoid contaminating the whole sample, pour a little urine on the test strip)
- send mid-stream urine (MSU) for culture if test positive or any urinary symptoms

Action	• ample fluid intake
	• rest
	• paracetamol/ibuprofen
	• assume a viral cause if no other clues, fever less than 1 week and generally well
	• otherwise give treatment appropriate to cause
	• explain that fever is produced by the body's immune system in response to an infection, is unlikely to cause any harm and may help recovery
Refer to GP	• immediately if:
	– over 1 week's duration
	– photophobia, neck stiffness, drowsiness, petechial rash
	– appears very unwell
	– travel to tropical area in last 3 months
Caution	• mastitis may cause 'flu-like symptoms in a breastfeeding woman with only minimal signs in the breast
	• malaria may cause an illness indistinguishable from 'flu (taking malaria prophylaxis may not prevent malaria)
	• meningitis in its early stages is impossible to distinguish from a simple viral infection. Ensure that the patient/parents know that they should phone again if symptoms worsen
	• fever with no associated other symptoms or signs of a focus of infection may require thorough investigation to discover the hidden cause

Hayfever

History	• April to August
	• frequent sneezing
	• blocked nose
	• red, itchy, watery eyes

- headache; dry, sore throat
- wheeze, chest tightness, cough
- has patient tried any over-the-counter treatment?
- with what effect?

Examination
- none

Tests
- none

Action
- advise patient:
  - to sleep with windows closed
  - to avoid long grass, fragrant flowers and newly mowed lawns

Prescription
- one or a combination of:
  - antihistamines: non-sedative, e.g. loratadine or fexo-fenadine, or sedative, e.g. chlorphen-iramine
  - eyedrops: sodium cromoglicate
  - nose spray: beclometasone aqueous nasal spray

Refer to GP
- if symptoms persist after various combinations of the above have been tried

Nosebleeds (epistaxis)

History
- duration
- extent of blood loss
- trauma, including nose-picking
- symptoms of sinusitis
- cold
- hayfever
- foreign body
- offensive discharge (may indicate a foreign body)

- previous episodes

- anaemia, leukaemia, anticoagulants

Examination
- which nostril?

- evidence of infection inside nostril?

- check blood pressure in adults

Tests
- consider FBC if severe/recurrent

Action
- advise pinching middle third of nose

- if infection seen, prescribe fusidic acid cream for 1 week

- if sinusitis present, refer to relevant section

Refer to GP
- urgently:

  - for referral to accident and emergency department if bleeding does not stop within 20 minutes

  - if blood disorder known or suspected, or patient is taking anticoagulants

- routinely:

  - if recurrent problem

- Herkner H, Laggner A, Mullner M *et al.* (2000) Hypertension in patients presenting with epistaxis. *Annals of Emergency Medicine.* **35**(2): 126–30.
- Ruddy J, Proops D, Pearman K *et al.* (1991) Management of epistaxis in children. *Int J Pediatr Otorhinolaryngol.* **21**: 139–42.

2 Head, neck and back

Headache

History
- duration
- onset (sudden/gradual/time of day/linked to menstrual cycle/linked to combined oral contraceptive)
- site on head
- associated symptoms:
  - visual disturbance
  - nausea
  - fever
  - cough
  - sinus problems
  - neck pain
- any known triggers
- previous recurrent headaches
- recent stress/worries/depression/disturbed sleep
- we all get headaches – what is different about this one?

Examination
- blood pressure (BP) (has to be really high – above 200/115 mmHg – to cause headache)
- tender sinuses (maxillary, frontal)
- neck movements/tenderness

Tests
- take blood for erythrocyte sedimentation rate (ESR) in patients over 60

Action
- reassure and explain, if cause is obvious
- suggest simple analgesics, e.g. co-codamol (paracetamol/codeine) or ibuprofen (most people have only tried paracetamol)

Refer to GP   • immediately if suspicious features:

  – sudden 'thunderclap' headache

  – other neurological symptoms

  – suspicion of meningitis

  – over 60

  – focal migraine in patient taking combined oral contraceptives

Caution   • temporal arteritis

  • meningitis

  • subarachnoid haemorrhage (sudden severe pain)

  } all very rare

Box 2.1   Temporal arteritis

This causes inflammation in small- to medium-sized arteries. It is more common over the age of 60. The headache is severe, often associated with tenderness of the scalp and sometimes aching of the jaw muscles on eating. There may be associated weakness of other muscles with morning stiffness, aches and weight loss.

It is significant because it may cause sudden occlusion of important blood vessels, resulting in blindness, stroke or myocardial infarction. A raised ESR will help in confirming the diagnosis. Long-term oral steroid treatment is needed.

Box 2.2   Migraine

Early symptoms such as excessive tiredness, yawning, pallor, visual disturbances and restlessness may start many hours before the headache. The headache is often severe, throbbing or bursting, unilateral, associated with nausea, and may last more than 24 h.

Migraine is caused by abnormal changes in the size of the blood vessels in the head and neck, although the initial event that starts an

continued

attack probably occurs in the brain, in the hypothalamus. A wide variety of factors are known to trigger migraine:

- stress
- light
- menstrual cycle hormones
- diet (caffeine, cheese, chocolate, citrus fruit, alcohol)
- starvation
- noise
- sleep disturbance
- hypoxia.

For most people the attacks seem to be multifactorial, and it is often not possible to identify any one trigger, which either always causes migraine or where avoidance stops all attacks. Whatever the cause, the final part of the sequence of events leading to symptoms involves the neurotransmitter 5-hydroxytryptamine (serotonin, 5-HT). Many new anti-migraine drugs are 5-HT agonists, which are used to treat attacks, not prevent them. Although these drugs are effective, they should only be prescribed when simpler and safer methods of treatment have failed.

Patients often know a remedy that works for them, for example a cup of tea, a lie-down in a quiet room and a short sleep. When this is either impractical or ineffective, then drugs have a role. Simple analgesics work for many sufferers, but they must be taken early in the attack. If there is associated nausea it is important to treat this as well, with an anti-emetic such as domperidone.

Migraine associated with difficulty in reading, particularly in children or young people, may respond to colour tinting of spectacles. Referral to an optometrist for an intuitive colorimeter test may both help the migraine and (importantly) improve educational potential.

If these measures do not control the migraine, refer to GP for consideration of specific anti-migraine therapy. If attacks are frequent (once a week) preventative treatment may be considered, although there is no ideal drug for this.

- Machlachlan A, Yale S and Wilkins A (1993) Open trial of subjective precision tinting: a follow-up of 55 patients. *Ophthal Physiol Optics.* **13**: 175–8.
- Ramadan NM, Schultz LL and Gilkey SJ (1987) Migraine prophylactic drugs: proof of efficacy, utilization and cost. *Cephalgia.* **17**: 73–80.

Notes on headache

Only about 10% of headaches have a treatable cause. Less than 0.5% are serious. Severe headaches are not necessarily the ones of greater concern. The commonest cause of headache is stress.

Table 2.1. Features of a suspicious headache

Reassuring	Suspicious
On the top of my head Like a band around my head It can last all day It can come on at any time I've had it for years on and off	Always there when I wake up Hurts more when I cough Localised Unilateral Sudden onset Associated with other symptoms: • visual, especially in elderly • nausea • weakness • numbness, pins and needles

Head injuries

History
- how did it happen?
- loss of consciousness
- confusion, convulsions, amnesia
- vomiting
- headache, drowsiness
- nervous system disturbance (e.g. numbness, paralysis, double vision)
- bleeding disorder, anticoagulants

Examination
- is the patient still confused or drowsy?
- look at injury
- check pupils:
  - are they equal?
  - do they react to light?
  - photophobia?

Tests
- none

Action
- give head injury instructions, if minor injury

Refer to GP
- immediately (for referral to hospital) if:
  - high-energy impact to head
  - loss of consciousness or amnesia
  - confusion
  - convulsions
  - vomiting
  - suspected skull fracture (orbital haematoma, deafness, clear cerebrospinal fluid from ear or nose)
  - alcohol intoxication
  - nervous system disturbance
  - unequal pupils
  - bleeding disorder or on anticoagulants
  - no-one to supervise patient at home

Box 2.3 Head injury instructions

Any injury or blow to the head will cause a certain degree of concussion. The seriousness of the concussion depends upon the severity of the injury. Nearly all patients with even slight concussion will probably have a headache for 48 h. They may well feel a little washed out and irritable during this period. Children often feel sick and may vomit once or twice and appear to be sleepy. This is to be expected in children who have had a blow to the head, and lasts 12–24 h.

Should
- the headache become severe
- the vomiting increase
- the sleepiness increase so that it is difficult to get the person to talk
- the irritability increase
- the person find that bright light in the eyes causes distress
- the person have a fit

then the person should be taken immediately to hospital for a further examination.

An adult with a suspected head injury should not return home alone. A child with a head injury should not be left unattended at home for any length of time. Simple paracetamol is suitable for pain relief.

continued overleaf

Advice to an adult after a head injury
- rest as much as possible, take a few days off work or study
- take paracetamol for headache
- avoid stress or major decisions
- avoid alcohol for a few days
- avoid driving alone or undertaking tiring journeys
- tell your employer or tutor that you have had a head injury
- return to work and routine daily activities gradually, avoiding overtime
- if you have problems which worry you or persist after 2 weeks, consult your doctor

After a head injury in a child
- allow the child to rest by reducing noise and light levels
- allow a few days off school
- give paracetamol for headache
- discourage noisy play or television programmes
- encourage plenty of drinks until normal appetite returns
- inform the teacher the child has had a head injury
- if your child has symptoms which worry you or persist after 2 weeks, consult your doctor

The above advice is based on head injury instructions from the Luton and Dunstable Hospital.

Dizziness

History
- duration
- nature: spinning (vertigo) or faint feeling
- associated symptoms:
  - nausea
  - earache
  - deafness
  - tinnitus
  - viral infection
- previous episodes
- medication (e.g. for BP)

Examination	• ears
	• BP (lying and standing in the elderly)
	• pale?
Tests	• FBC if anaemia suspected
	• otherwise none
Advice	• dizziness is common, often accompanies viral infections
	• will usually settle, but may sometimes take several weeks
	• sit and stand slowly; rest
Prescription	• if true vertigo, prochlorperazine
Refer to GP	• urgently if:
	– neurological symptoms/signs
	– headache
	– deafness, especially if new and unilateral
	– previous ear surgery
	– previous recent head injury
	• routinely if:
	– on treatment and BP is low
	– persistent/recurrent symptoms

Neck pain

History	• duration
	• injury, e.g. whiplash
	• sore throat
	• is patient worried about meningitis?

- occupation (e.g. seamstress, keyboard operator)
- onset: sudden/known trigger/gradual

Examination
- cervical lymph nodes
- neck movement and their limits
- posture

Tests
- none

Action
- analgesia, e.g. ibuprofen or paracetamol
- local heat
- gentle exercises – give leaflet
- attention to posture
- reassure not meningitis

Refer to GP
- if severe pain, or not responding to simple analgesics in 4–5 days

Caution
- instantaneous onset of neck pain and stiffness may be due to subarachnoid haemorrhage

Back pain

History
- occupation
- gradual/sudden onset
- while lifting?
- duration/previous episodes
- radiation to legs – below knee?
- numbness/tingling of legs or perianal area?
- difficulty passing urine?

Examination
- ask patient to show site of pain
- spinal movement (flexion/extension/rotation)
- straight leg raising – record angles

Tests   • not necessary

Action   • reassure the patient that most back pain is not serious and will get better without treatment

                 • encourage gentle mobilisation (activity within the limits of pain as soon as possible)

                 • if pain is very severe recommend lying flat on the floor or firm bed, for 2–3 days at the most

                 • analgesics relieve pain and muscle spasm:

                   – ibuprofen

                   – paracetamol

                   – co-codamol

                 • short courses of these drugs are cheaper if bought over the counter

                 • give back care leaflet

                 • recommend manipulation if available/affordable

Refer to GP   • **urgently** if numbness/tingling in perianal area or difficulty passing urine (both extremely rare)

                 • **urgently** if sudden onset of severe pain with stiffness and no apparent cause

                 • make appointment if severe symptoms or sciatica (pain/numbness/tingling in one leg extending below the knee)

                 • if elderly or taking oral corticosteroids

Caution   • unilateral pain over renal area may have a renal cause: arrange urine dipstick test and MSU for culture

                 • instantaneous onset of back pain and stiffness without an obvious trigger may be due to subarachnoid haemorrhage

                 • back pain may be caused by abdominal pathology such as an aortic aneurysm

• Managing acute low back pain (1998) *Drug Therap Bull.* **36**(12): 93–5.

3 Eyes and skin

Sore eyes

History
- duration
- contact (e.g. sibling)
- associated cold symptoms
- any problem with vision?
- history of foreign body
- discharge
- contact lens use

Examination
- discharge
- redness
- one/both sides
- pupils equal and react to light
- visual acuity (may be omitted in cases of simple conjunctivitis when the patient has reported no change in vision)
- look for foreign body (evert eyelid) if symptoms unilateral
- painful clusters of spots around eye (possible shingles)

Tests
- take swab if persistent or recurrent symptoms
- stain with fluorescein if unilateral/history of trauma/recent use of power tools

Action
1 Infective conjunctivitis
(sore eyes, red conjunctival membranes with or without pus)

- administer chloramphenicol eyedrops as often as possible (every hour or so ideally); if severe, apply ointment at night also (suitable for all ages; treat only the infected eye(s))
- if contact lenses are worn, suggest that they are cleaned and not used until the eye has healed

- warn – contagious

- use own face cloth and towel

- schools and nurseries prefer that children with conjunctivitis do not attend

2 Allergic conjunctivitis
(longer history, less angry inflammation, frequent 'attacks', no pus)

- avoid trigger, e.g. make-up

- if prescription needed, sodium cromoglicate drops four times a day

3 Dry eyes
(elderly usually affected, eyes feel gritty but look normal, vision unaffected)

- artificial tears help if used often (hypromellose, available over the counter)

Refer to GP
- same day if:

    - abnormal shape or reaction of pupils to light

    - reduced visual acuity, blurred vision

    - foreign body in eye or under eyelid

    - persistent/recurrent symptoms

    - severe inflammation

    - shingles suspected

    - any abnormality seen using fluorescein

Caution
- iritis (not all conjunctival area red, unequal/irregular pupils, photophobia)

- glaucoma (pain in eye, decrease in visual acuity)

- *Chlamydia* (pale bumps on inner lids)

- herpes (cold sores, shingles)

- contact lens problems (consult optometrist)

Subconjunctival haemorrhage

This may sometimes be confused with conjunctivitis. It causes a sudden uniform red area in the eye with a sharp edge. You should be able to see the posterior margin. There is no discomfort, discharge or deterioration in vision. Patients often worry that the haemorrhage may be a sign of high BP. Although there is no evidence for this, checking the BP will reassure the patient.

Styes

History
- how long present?
- has it discharged?

Examination
- any associated conjunctivitis?

Tests
- none

Action
- none may be necessary if resolving or discharged
- otherwise give chloramphenicol eye ointment
- warn that styes are infectious; care with hygiene
- if there is any sign of cellulitis of the eyelid, give antibiotics (*see* page 49)

Rashes

History
- duration
- did all spots appear at same time, or gradually?
- fever/malaise
- spots, or weals which come and go?
- any contacts who are itching?
- pregnant?
- on any medication?

Examination	• site and distribution (remember to look in the mouth)
	• are the spots clearly defined and separate?
	• or weal-like (irregular, raised, blotchy)?
	• flat (macules) or raised (papules)?
	• are there burrows on the hands?
	• are there blisters? Large or small?
Tests	• none
Action/referral	• see different diagnoses

Acute itchy rashes

Acute itchy rashes may be caused by:

• chickenpox
• urticaria
• scabies
• eczema (*see* page 39)
• fungal infections (*see* page 42)

Chickenpox

• separate itchy papules at different stages of development
• turning to blisters
• fever and malaise, more marked in adults

Action	• calamine lotion OTC (keep in fridge)
	• perhaps antihistamines – chlorpheniramine is useful for children at night because of its sedative action
	• inform contacts who are pregnant, on steroids or immuno-suppressed

Refer to GP   • urgently if:

                  – on steroids

                  – immunosuppressed, e.g. transplant patients, HIV

                  – breathless

                  – confused/severe headache

                  – pregnant

                  – less than 4 weeks after childbirth

                  – a baby aged under 4 weeks

Urticaria

- also called 'nettle rash'
- raised irritating weals
- no other symptoms
- may be due to drugs (e.g. aspirin, antibiotics) or food allergy
- or reaction to heat or sunlight, hot bath or vigorous exercise
- or reaction to pressure or cold
- or may be viral

Action   • oral (not topical) antihistamines:

                  – chlorpheniramine if sedation is acceptable

                  – loratadine or fexofenadine if sedation is not acceptable

Refer to GP   • if drug allergy suspected

Scabies

- spreading variable rash
- widespread itching, worse at night
- rash never found on face
- burrows may be visible on hands, or elsewhere
- sleeping partners or other family members may be affected

Action
- malathion aqueous lotion
- antihistamines (as above)
- stress that *itching may persist for several weeks* after mites have been eradicated

A rash in a seriously ill patient

A rash in a seriously ill patient may be caused by:

- measles
- meningococcal septicaemia

Measles

- extremely rare nowadays
- a severe respiratory infection
- cough
- conjunctivitis
- bright red flat areas which coalesce, mainly on trunk

Action
- complete 'notification of infectious diseases' form
- check for otitis media

Meningococcal septicaemia

- extremely rare but very important
- patient looks ill, often drowsy or confused
- fever
- diarrhoea is a common early feature
- rash is purpuric (i.e. dull red, does not blanch on pressure using a glass)

Refer to GP
- *immediately* for an injection of benzyl penicillin and transfer to hospital by emergency ambulance

A rash in a mildly febrile patient

A rash in a mildly febrile patient may be caused by:

- rubella
- parvovirus
- hand, foot and mouth disease
- roseola infantum
- streptococcal infection

Rubella

Many viruses cause a diffuse macular rash. Experts get this wrong frequently – safest to say 'it's a virus'; after all, rubella is a virus!

- check for pharyngitis (*see* page 38)

Action
- inform pregnant contacts
- no treatment needed

Refer to GP
- if pregnant

Parvovirus

- 'slapped cheeks'
- diffuse macular rash
- cold symptoms
- joint pains in adults

Action
- no treatment needed

Refer to GP
- if pregnant (may cause miscarriage)

Hand, foot and mouth disease

- caused by a virus
- blisters on hands, feet and in mouth

- fever and malaise

- not related to foot and mouth disease in animals

Action   • no treatment needed

Roseola infantum

- in infants

- fever for a few days

- then rose pink maculopapular rash on neck and trunk

- no treatment needed

Streptococcal infection

- generalised macular rash

- sore throat/tonsillitis

- cervical lymphadenopathy

- fever and malaise

Action   • antibiotic recommended (*see* page 1)

Other rashes

Other rashes may be caused by:

- impetigo

- eczema

- shingles

- pityriasis rosea

- fungal infections

Impetigo

- golden crusted lesions
- commonly on faces of children, though may occur elsewhere
- topical fusidic acid if mild
- oral flucloxacillin if severe (erythromycin if the patient is allergic to penicillin)
- off school for 2 days
- use own face cloth and towel

Eczema

History
- duration
- previous episodes
- suspected cause (e.g. solvents, metals, soap, latex)
- itch
- discharge
- what treatment has been tried?
- distribution

Examination
- look at offending area
- is it infected/inflamed/weeping?

Tests
- swab if discharging
- scrapings for fungus (if diagnosis in doubt, or treatment unsuccessful)

Action
- emollients and bath additives, e.g. emulsifying ointment, hydrous ointment, Oilatum emollient (or ask pharmacist)
- topical steroid creams (1% hydrocortisone initially)
- avoid detergents (e.g. bubble bath)

- if hands affected use cotton-lined rubber gloves for washing-up

- antibiotics if infected (topical fusidic acid or oral flucloxacillin, or erythromycin if allergic to penicillin)

Refer to GP • if vesicles or severe infection

Caution • *fungal infection* may look very similar but is usually asymmetrical

- *infection* is common, usually with *Staphylococcus aureus*. May cause a sudden flare of angry, itchy eczema or an impetigo-like rash. Use topical fusidic acid or oral flucloxacillin (erythromycin if the patient is allergic to penicillin)

- *Herpes simplex* may produce vesicles or chickenpox-like areas. Refer to GP if suspected

Notes on eczema

- common

- may be general tendency in atopic individuals or localised in response to insult to skin

- dry, cracking, sore

- cure impossible except in acute, short-lived cases:

  - diets
  - herbal tea
  - acupuncture
  - application of urine

  are little help, even though people put faith in them hoping to find a cure

- reducing exposure to house dust mite may help (e.g. anti-allergenic mattress and pillow covers, wooden floors and the use of vacuum cleaners with anti-allergenic filters)

- control is the aim, using frequent application of emollients (e.g. emulsifying ointment) to rehydrate the skin and prevent evaporation from the surface.

Topical steroids stronger than hydrocortisone may cause atrophy and thinning of the skin after prolonged use. Tiny blood vessels become visible, for which no treatment is available. The skin of the face is the most sensitive, the palms and soles least sensitive. Children's skin is more sensitive than adults' – **do not use anything stronger than hydrocortisone in children, or on the face**.

Table 3.1. Creams and ointments for eczema

Preparation	Potency	Maximum use
Betnovate	High	6 weeks
Eumovate	Moderate	8 weeks
Hydrocortisone	Low	12 weeks to indefinitely
Emollients	Zero	Indefinitely
Bath additives	Zero	Indefinitely

• Using topical corticosteroids in general practice (1999) *MeReC Bull.* **10**(6): 21–4.

Nappy rash

History	• duration
	• creams tried
Examination	• mild/severe
	• satellite spots
	• involving skin creases
Tests	• none
Action	• frequent nappy changes
	• leave nappy off when possible
	• avoid plastic pants
	• if using washable nappies, care in sterilising/rinsing and consider using disposables

- reassure parent that some children are simply prone to nappy rash

Prescription
- if fungal infection suspected (satellite spots/creases involved) use clotrimazole cream and barrier cream

- if mild, advise barrier cream, e.g. zinc and castor oil

- if severe, use miconazole/hydrocortisone ointment for 1 week only and barrier cream on top (may need further antifungal after miconazole hydrocortisone finished)

Refer to GP
- if not responding to treatment, or consider health visitor referral

Fungal infections

- of the foot (athlete's foot)
- flexures
- body ('ringworm')

History
- itchy rash, slowly spreading
- not usually symmetrical

Examination
- eczema-like patches
- often a scaly, inflamed edge
- central area may appear normal
- in toe webs, under breasts

Action
- explain that it is an infection acquired from other humans or animals
- keep as dry as possible

Prescription
- clotrimazole cream for 3 weeks

Refer to GP
- if it persists despite an adequate course of treatment

Cold sores

History	• often recurrent on same site
	• tingling in skin before appearance of the sore
	• current or preceding febrile illness?
	• exposure to strong sunlight?
	• stress or other psychological trigger?
Examination	• itchy, sore cluster of small blisters on a red patch, most commonly on the lips, but may be on the face, inside the mouth, or sometimes on genitalia
Tests	• none
Action	• aciclovir cream if within 48 h of appearance (not in pregnancy)
	• advise those working with babies under 6 months that they should not work until the sore has healed (*herpes simplex* can cause a very serious illness in small babies)
	• take care not to touch eyes after touching cold sore
Refer to GP	• if recurrent
Caution	• secondary bacterial infection of cold sore, causing yellow crusting and cellulitis (*see* Impetigo, page 39)
	• beware of the very rare eczema herpeticum, a wide-spread eruption in a person with atopic eczema; can be life-threatening

• Worrell G (1991) Topical acyclovir for recurrent herpes labialis in primary care. *Can Fam Phys.* **37**: 92–8 (abstract in the Cochrane Library).

Genital herpes

History
- intensely painful ulcers or blisters on the genitalia
- may be recurrent

Refer to GP
- always; referral to genitourinary clinic may be necessary

Shingles

History
- discomfort or pain often starts up to 5 days before the rash
- affects the area of skin supplied by one nerve root (*see* Figure 3.1)
- therefore only one side of the body is affected
- malaise, mild fever
- may start after a period of debility
- previous history of chickenpox
- commoner and more likely to cause long-term pain in the elderly

Examination
- painful blisters in the area of skin supplied by one nerve root (dermatome)
- some may weep fluid (which is infectious)
- note which nerve root is affected (*see* Figure 3.1)
- if the face is affected, does the rash involve the forehead, cheek or the tip of the nose? Is the eye red?
- local lymph nodes may be enlarged

Tests
- none

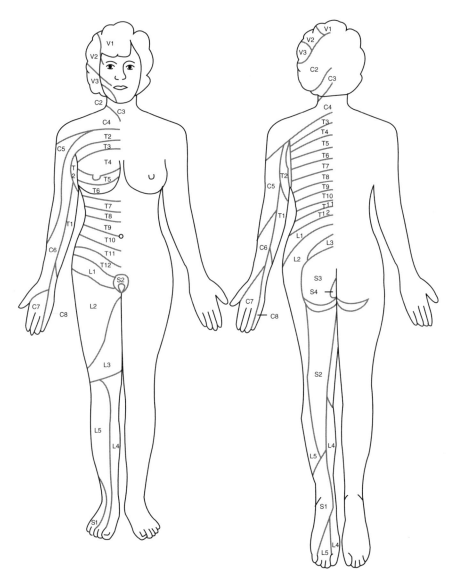

Figure 3.1 Dermatome diagram. Each area is labelled with the spinal nerve that carries sensation from the skin to the spinal cord. The areas overlap to some extent, and an individual person may vary from normal. C, cervical; L, lumbar; S, sacral; T, thoracic; V, fifth cranial nerve (trigeminal).

Action
- explain the diagnosis:
  - the rash will dry within 1 week
- advise:
  - keep the rash dry
  - avoid contact with newborn infants, pregnant women or people who are ill or infirm
  - a patient with chickenpox or shingles may infect someone else with chickenpox, but not with shingles
  - creams and lotions are of little or no help and best avoided because of the risk of spreading skin bacteria into the blistered area
  - seek medical advice again if the rash 'flares up' (because of secondary infection)
  - malaise may require rest and time off work
- ibuprofen or co-codamol for pain

Refer to GP
- if face or eye affected (see above)
- anyone who is unwell with a concurrent illness, e.g. cancer
- if the pain is troublesome despite simple analgesia
- if aged over 75

- Lancaster T, Silagy C and Gray S (1995) Primary care management of acute herpes zoster: systematic review of evidence from randomised controlled trials. *Br J Gen Pract.* **45**: 39–45 (reviewed in *Bandolier* 1995, **17**: 3).

Pityriasis rosea

History
- an acute eruption of numerous, widespread, pink, scaly, oval patches 1–4 cm in diameter, occurring over a period of days
- usually a larger initial 'herald' patch
- the patches often follow the skin creases and mainly affect the trunk, face, scalp and limbs

- there may be itching, usually mild but occasionally intense

- it occurs mainly in adolescents and young adults, and more often during autumn or spring

- there may have been malaise, fever or lymphadenopathy before the rash appeared

Tests
- none

Action
- no treatment is required

- the rash will last 6–10 weeks then disappear, leaving no trace

- explain the condition and its course to the patient and reassure that it is not contagious, nor does it recur

Warts and verrucae

Examination
- raised pale bumps, or flattened areas with black dots on soles of feet

Explain
- caused by a virus

- most disappear by themselves with time, but may take years

- contagious

Action

Options:

1 Leave alone

2 Soak in warm water for 5 minutes twice daily, remove dead skin with an emery board, then apply glutaraldehyde. Persevere until completely disappeared; may take 3 months

3 Liquid nitrogen – not for children under the age of 10 as can be painful. Can also cause dramatic blood blistering, temporary numbness and a scar

Even vigorous procedures do not always succeed and warts often reappear at the treated site. A patient with a verruca should use a waterproof plaster or verruca sock for swimming and PE and avoid sharing a towel.

Refer to GP
- anogenital warts
- single warts in the elderly (may be a squamous carcinoma)

Molluscum contagiosum

Molluscum contagiosum is a poxvirus infection which produces clusters of round, raised, pearly white lesions (sometimes with a darker central dimple) on the trunk and limbs of children. It is best left untreated as it resolves completely, without scarring, after several months.

Boils

History
- duration
- fever
- thirst/polyuria/tiredness
- predisposing factors (diabetes, steroids, immuno-suppression)

Examination
- cellulitis
- enlarged lymph nodes
- pallor

Tests
- if recurrent boils, or symptoms or family history of diabetes, test blood glucose and FBC

Action
- apply heat to encourage pointing
- magnesium sulphate paste is traditionally used, although there is no evidence to support it

- if cellulitis, fever or severe pain:

  – flucloxacillin for 7 days

  – erythromycin if the patient is allergic to penicillin

Refer to GP
- urgently if facial boil causing cellulitis (can be life-threatening), or boil in anogenital area or natal cleft (between buttocks)

- make appointment if recurrent boils

Infected wounds/cellulitis

History
- duration

- nature of wound

- fever/malaise

- tetanus status

- altered immunity (diabetes, taking corticosteroids or other immunosuppressants)

Examination
- discharge

- cellulitis

- lymphadenopathy

Tests
- take swabs if discharge from a significant wound

- blood glucose if history of recurrent skin infections

Action
- wound cleaning and dressing as appropriate

- fusidic acid ointment for mild superficial infections

- oral flucloxacillin for 7 days for more severe infections (erythromycin if the patient is allergic to penicillin)

- if deeper cellulitis is present, add amoxicillin to flucloxacillin or use co-amoxiclav (erythromycin if the patient is allergic to penicillin)

- tetanus booster if due

Refer to GP	• same day if:

       – diabetic/altered immunity

       – severe infection

       – pointing abscess (for incision and drainage)

       – in anogenital area or natal cleft (between buttocks)

Ingrowing toenail

History	• duration
	• discharge
	• previous episodes
	• diabetes
Examination	• cellulitis
	• discharge
	• granulation
Tests	• swab if discharge
Action	• advise to insert a pledget of cotton wool to lift the corner of nail away from the flesh
	• chiropody referral if persistent/recurrent
	• if localised cellulitis, give flucloxacillin for 7 days (or erythromycin if allergic to penicillin)
Caution	• risk of severe foot infection in patients with diabetes

• Ingrowing toenail treatments (1999) *Bandolier.* **69**(11): 1–2.
• Connolly B and Fitzgerald R (1988) Pledgets in ingrowing toenails. *Arch Dis Child.* **63**(1): 71–2.

Head lice

History	• nits
	• lice
	• scratching

Examination	• examine head
	• may have enlarged lymph nodes at back of neck
	• nits (louse eggs adhere to hair tightly, whereas dandruff falls off easily)
	• examination unnecessary if parent sure of diagnosis
Tests	• none
Action	• follow current local recommendations
	• check all of household and treat **affected people only** (repeat after 2 weeks)
	• apply conditioner liberally, then use fine metal comb to break the legs of the lice, so that they cannot reproduce
	• reassure – lice prefer clean hair
	• warn patient that eggs will be visible after treatment
Refer to GP	• or health visitor if recurrent problems
Caution	• those with asthma should use *aqueous* malathion and avoid alcoholic lotions which can cause wheezing

• Management of head louse infection (1999) *Prescribing Nurse Bull.* **1**(4): 13–16.

Moles

Most moles develop in early childhood and adolescence, and there is a gradual decrease in their number in old age. Not unreasonably, malignant melanoma is a concern behind many consultations, in which most patients need reassurance.

History	• patient's concern about the mole
	• increase in size?
	• change in colour or shape?

Examination	• there are seven points to look for and ask about:

  1 size – most benign moles are less than 1 cm in diameter. Any increase?

  2 shape – has it a regular, well-defined edge?

  3 colour – is colour even throughout? Any change?

  4 itching

  5 bleeding

  6 crusting

  7 inflammation

Tests
• none

Action
• reassure if two or fewer of the above seven points are true, in which case the mole is almost certainly not a malignant melanoma

• advise:

  – on the points above

  – to watch the mole themselves; maybe measure it or trace its outline, and come back if it is enlarging

  – to take a sensible approach to sun exposure

Refer to GP
• if:

  – more than two of the above seven points are true

  – any mole has been increasing in size and is now over 0.5 cm in diameter

  – any change in shape or colour

Caution
• many so-called moles are, in fact, seborrhoeic keratoses (senile warts), which are golden brown in colour with a scaly, greasy surface. They are harmless

• beware slowly growing, ulcerated or raised areas with a raised edge. They may be skin carcinomas: basal cell carcinomas (rodent ulcers) are commonly found on the faces and foreheads of elderly people

• Mackie R, Doherty V, Keefe M *et al.* (1991) Seven-point checklist for melanoma. *Clin Experi Derm.* **16**(2): 151–3.

Insect bites and stings

History
- site
- nature of insect, if known
- problem in previous years?

Examination
- size of reaction
- is sting still *in situ* (rare)?

Tests
- none

Action
- 1% hydrocortisone cream
- oral antihistamine, e.g. loratadine or fexofenadine
- avoid topical antihistamines, which are not effective and may themselves cause irritation

Refer to GP
- urgently if:
  - swelling of lips or tongue
  - anaphylactic shock (extremely rare)

Caution
- it may sometimes be difficult to distinguish allergy from infection, which usually develops after 24 h and becomes progressively worse
- recurrent bites on the legs are usually due to dog or cat fleas in carpets or rugs

Sunburn

History
- duration of exposure
- sunscreens

Examination
- extent of burn
- blistering

Tests	• none
Action	• safe sun advice
	• leave blisters intact if possible
Prescription	• hydrocortisone cream 2.5%
	• in adults, if severe, Betnovate cream for a few days

• Russo P and Schneiderman L (1978) Effect of topical corticosteroids on symptoms of clinical sunburn. *J Fam Pract.* **7**(6): 1129–32.

Mouth problems

Oral candidiasis (thrush)

A fungal infection, common in babies, those using inhaled corticosteroids and those whose immunity is poor.

History	• soreness
	• difficulty in eating/drinking
Examination	• white patches on tongue and oral mucosa that cannot easily be removed
Tests	• mouth swab may be useful if the diagnosis is in doubt
Action/ prescription	• nystatin oral suspension or miconazole gel (OTC)
	• for those using inhaled steroids, ensure that spacer is used and recommend that after use they gargle with water and then spit it out

Aphthous ulcers

History	• painful ulcers
	• may occur anywhere in the mouth, most commonly on the buccal mucosa (lining of the cheek)

Examination	• red, round lesions, sometimes with white crater
Action/ prescription	• Adcortyl in Orabase may help the pain
Refer to GP	• if persisting/enlarging ulcer (may be a carcinoma)

Hand, foot and mouth disease

See page 37.

Herpes simplex stomatitis

As well as the familiar cold sore (*see* page 43) the *herpes simplex* virus may cause a systemic illness with extensive ulceration of the mouth when it is first encountered.

History	• usually a small child
	• short history of fever and malaise
	• refusing to eat or drink
Examination	• dehydration
	• multiple small ulcers on tongue, palate and buccal mucosa (cheek lining)
Action	• ensure adequate fluid intake (a straw or very cold drinks may help)
Refer to GP	• urgently if symptoms of less than 48 hours' duration, for consideration of oral aciclovir

• Amir J, Harel L, Smetana Z *et al.* (1997) Treatment of *herpes simplex* gingivostomatitis with aciclovir in children: a randomised double-blind placebo controlled study. *BMJ.* **314**: 1800–3 (reviewed in *Evidence-based Medicine.* 1998, **Jan/Feb**: 6).

Dental infections

History	• site of pain
	• swelling

- fever

- duration

- when dentist last consulted

Examination
- record site of pain/swelling

- obvious dental decay

Action
- advise seeing dentist within 1 week

- give antibiotics and painkillers, if your practice agrees: some have a policy not to provide treatment for dental problems

Prescription
- metronidazole for 5 days (amoxicillin if the patient is sensitive to metronidazole)

- treatment with an appropriate antibiotic usually provides rapid relief of pain, but if additional analgesia is required suggest ibuprofen or paracetamol. Avoid dihydrocodeine, which may make dental pain worse

- Seymour RA, Rawlins MD and Rowell FJ (1982) Dihydrocodeine-induced hyperalgesia in postoperative dental pain. *Lancet.* **1**(8287): 1425–6.

4 Abdomen

Abdominal pain

History
- site
- duration
- intermittent/continuous
- stabbing/dull/colicky
- previous episodes (diagnosis and outcome)
- previous abdominal operations
- associated features:
  - fever
  - constipation/diarrhoea
  - vomiting/nausea/anorexia
  - dysuria/frequency
  - pain in testicles or groin
  - date of last menstrual period (LMP)/vaginal discharge/contraception
  - upper respiratory tract infection in children (may cause abdominal pain due to enlarged lymph nodes)

Examination
- examine abdomen
- record site of pain, any tenderness
- examine tonsils in children

Tests
- test urine for protein/blood/glucose/nitrites (write result in notes)
- MSU for culture if urinary symptoms

Refer to GP
- always, unless obvious gastroenteritis or urinary tract infection (UTI) (*see* those protocols)

- urgently if:

  - severe

  - less than 1 week history

  - testicular or groin pain

Caution
- *Ectopic pregnancy* causes severe lower abdominal pain, usually one-sided, in a woman whose period is late or just due. She may collapse with the pain, particularly if a vaginal examination is attempted. If suspected, refer to GP urgently

Indigestion

History
- site of pain/discomfort

- heartburn

- relation to meals

- relation to exercise

- smoking

- alcohol

- consumption of large amounts of particular foods (e.g. fried foods, orange juice, curries)

- stress

- associated symptoms:

  - vomiting

  - weight loss

- previous episodes, how treated

- drugs, especially aspirin, non-steroidal anti-inflammatory drugs (NSAIDs)

Examination
- feel abdomen

- record site of pain

Tests	• none
Action	• stop any NSAID
	• only stop aspirin if it is being taken for pain
	• advise antacids initially, e.g. magnesium trisilicate
	• cimetidine if these have been tried and are ineffective
	• change of diet
Prescription	• magnesium trisilicate (or recommend purchase over the counter, if patient pays prescription charges)
	• cimetidine for 7 days (check if on any other medication and any drug interactions)
Refer to GP	• urgently if:
	– sudden onset or related to exercise (may be cardiac)
	– vomiting, weight loss
	• routinely if:
	– aged over 45
	– persistent/recurrent symptoms
	– patient has been taking regular NSAID or aspirin

Diarrhoea and vomiting

History	• duration: preceding constipation?
	• severity: number of episodes in last 24 h
	• blood (red or black) in motion/vomit
	• fever
	• contacts with similar symptoms
	• foreign travel
	• suspect meals
	• occupation – food handler?

- in children: adequate urine output?
- history of bowel disease
- relevant medication (e.g. antibiotics or NSAIDs)

Examination
- dehydration
- fontanelle in babies under 1 year
- dry tongue/mouth
- dry skin not reshaping after a soft pinch
- dry eyes, no tears, not reflecting light
- consider rectal examination if overflow suspected (*see* Caution)

Test
- stool culture if:
  - suspicion of food poisoning
  - blood in motion
  - recent travel to countries with poor hygiene
  - symptoms for 5 days or more
    - (i)   collect 5 ml sample from potty/chamberpot, or put clingfilm on the toilet
    - (ii) put name on bottle
    - (iii) complete bacteriology form
- also MSU in children under 5 with persistent or recurrent diarrhoea or vomiting

Action
- reassurance: rarely serious
- dehydration is rare over 6 months of age
  - explain warning signs
- recommend washing hands after using toilet
- food handlers should not work until symptoms settle
- small frequent sips of clear fluids for 12 h, for example:
  - flat, cold cola (good for vomiting children)
  - apple juice
  - Dioralyte only for babies under 6 months of age

- after 12 h progress to high-calorie, low-fibre, milk-free diet, e.g. jelly, clear soup, bread and spread, boiled rice

Prescription
- paracetamol for stomach cramps

- loperamide if diarrhoea is disabling (over 12 years only)

- kaolin preparations are useless

- adult patients who are very unwell or socially devastated by their symptoms could be offered:

  - buccal prochlorperazine (for vomiting in those over 20 years)

  - domperidone (for vomiting in teenagers – consider suppositories or injection if vomiting is severe)

Notification
- notify immediately if food poisoning suspected because of the history or symptom of bloody diarrhoea or if confirmed by culture. Complete form from *Notification of Infectious Diseases* book. Tell patients that someone from the Public Health Department may contact them

Refer to GP
- urgently:

  - those with diabetes

  - those with inflammatory bowel disease (ulcerative colitis or Crohn's)

  - those with diverticular disease

  - if symptoms are side effects of a drug which will need to be changed (urgency of referral depends on why the drug was prescribed)

  - if severely ill/dehydrated

  - if blood (red or brown) in vomit

  - if significant blood (red or black) in stools

  - if severe diarrhoea and malaise, for consideration of quinolone (e.g. ciprofloxacin) therapy

Caution
- spurious or 'overflow' diarrhoea may be caused by severe constipation. If in doubt, do a rectal examination

- diarrhoea is a common early feature of meningococcal septicaemia

- gastrointestinal side effects from drugs are common especially if the patient has recently started an analgesic or an antibiotic

- Farthing M, Feldman R, Finch R *et al.* (1996) The management of infective gastroenteritis in adults. A consensus statement by an expert panel convened by the British Society for the Study of Infection. *J Infect.* **33**: 143–52.
- Murphy M (1998) Guidelines for managing acute gastroenteritis based on a systematic review of published research. *Arch Dis Child.* **79**: 279–84.

Constipation

History	- duration; habitual?
	- how often bowels open?
	- consistency of motion/straining
	- blood in motion or on the toilet paper?
	- abdominal pain
	- vomiting
	- previous abdominal operations
	- changes in weight
	- medication (e.g. analgesics containing codeine)
Examination	- usually none
	- consider rectal examination if diagnosis/severity in doubt
Tests	- none
Action	- more fluids
	- high-fibre diet
	- review drugs – on codeine preparations?
	- lactulose (mild) or senna (severe)
	- may need to continue treatment for several weeks
	- in emergencies, glycerol suppositories

Refer to GP   • urgently if:

- associated with vomiting and/or previous abdominal operation

• routinely if:

- sudden change in bowel habit, weight loss or rectal bleeding in adults

- symptoms persist or treatment is still necessary after 1 week in children

Rectal problems

Box 4.1   Rectal problems

Haemorrhoids ('piles')

These are distended veins inside the anal canal, which have a similar appearance to varicose veins. They may prolapse ('come down') on straining, when they may be visible as soft, purple grape-like swellings protruding from the anus. They may cause bleeding, itching or discomfort.

Thrombosed external pile

This is caused by a sudden leakage of blood from a small blood vessel near the anus. The blood stretches the sensitive skin and is very painful. It will gradually disperse, but if the patient presents early it is possible to incise it and relieve pain by releasing the blood clot.

Anal fissure

A split in the anal skin, usually caused by passing a large, hard stool. This is a common cause of pain and bleeding on defecation. Most will heal within 6 weeks, provided that the stools remain soft.

History	• bleeding on defecation:
	  – how much? In toilet pan/on paper only?
	  – bright red/dark red
	• pain on defecation
	• itch (threadworms)
	• swelling near anus? Does a swelling appear on straining?
	• constipation

Examination	• any visible swelling? • any split in perianal skin?

Action	• advise:
	  – avoid straining – laxatives
	  – high-fibre diet
	  – alternate wet/dry toilet tissue
	  – sit on bag of frozen peas wrapped in a towel if the discomfort is severe

Prescription	• consider lactulose short term • high-fibre diet • emulsifying ointment or Anusol cream, or Xyloproct if pain is severe

Refer to GP	• urgently if:
	  – severe bleeding
	  – dark blood (may come from a carcinoma high inside the bowel)
	• routinely if:
	  – persistent or recurrent problems

Caution	• remember the possibility of sexual abuse or sexually transmitted diseases

Urinary tract infection/cystitis

History
- duration
- dysuria/frequency
- obvious haematuria
- fever/abdominal pain/vomiting
- loin pain
- vaginal discharge
- recurrent symptoms
- associated with intercourse (NB teenagers may need contraception)
- possibility of pregnancy?
- previous history of renal stones or pyelonephritis

Examination
- in small boys check the penis for redness (*see* balanitis, page 67)

Tests
- urinalysis for blood/protein, nitrites, if urine readily available (to avoid contaminating the whole sample, pour a little urine on to the test strip)
- MSU *before starting treatment* in:
  - children (bag or pad samples may be needed in infants)
  - men
  - pregnant women
  - those with persistent recurrent symptoms
  - those with fever/loin pain

  and arrange follow-up MSU after treatment (unnecessary for uncomplicated UTI in women)
- if associated vaginal discharge:
  - high vaginal and cervical swabs for culture and *Chlamydia* test

Action
- high fluid intake
- cranberry juice
- patient to phone for MSU results (if applicable)

Prescription
- antibiotics:

  - uncomplicated UTI in non-pregnant women: trimethoprim for 3 days
    or
    nitrofurantoin MR for 3 days (depending on local patterns of antibiotic resistance)

  - children or men: trimethoprim for 7 days (or cefalexin for 7 days if allergic to trimethoprim)

  - pregnant women: cefalexin for 7 days

  - fever/loin pain/previous pyelonephritis: cefalexin for 7 days

Refer to GP
- urgently if high fever/loin pain/severe pain/malaise

  - history of kidney stones/pyelonephritis

- routinely (when UTI confirmed by MSU result) in:

  - children (urine infections may cause kidney damage)

  - men

  - women with severe/persistent symptoms

  - patients with loin pain

- in children, do not wait for the MSU result before starting antibiotics

Caution
- some women confuse the symptoms of thrush and cystitis

- *Chlamydia* infections may cause dysuria

- The management of urinary tract infection in children (1997) *Drug Therap Bull.* **35**(9): 65–9.

Threadworms

History
- perianal irritation

- anal pain at night

- worms may be seen – like white cotton threads – on skin or in stool

Examination	• not necessary

Tests	• tests are not necessary unless the diagnosis is in doubt. Sellotape applied to the anus first thing in the morning will pick up the eggs. Stick the sellotape on to a microscope slide labelled with the patient's name and send it to the Public Health Laboratory for confirmation of the diagnosis

Action	• an appointment is not necessary if the parent is sure of the diagnosis
	• explain that adult threadworms live for only 6 weeks – their eggs must be transferred to the mouth and swallowed for the infection to continue
	• as well as the prescription, hygienic measures are necessary:

  – wash hands and scrub nails before each meal and after going to the toilet

  – bathe in early morning to remove eggs laid during the night

  – change bed linen

  – cut fingernails

Treatment	• mebendazole for adults (unless pregnant or breast-feeding) and children over 2 years
	• piperazine for children under 2 years and infection in pregnant or lactating women
	• treat all members of household

• Threadworms (1999) *Presc Nurse Bull.* **1**(3): 11–12.

Balanitis (sore penis)

History	• duration
	• swelling of foreskin
	• discharge

- dysuria
- previous episodes

Examination
- gently attempt to retract foreskin in boys aged 3 and over
- localised redness
- or generalised cellulitis

Tests
- swab if discharge
- MSU for culture if no redness visible

Action
- advise gentle cleaning under foreskin in boys aged 3 and over (ensure it is pulled down afterwards)
- if difficulty in passing urine because of pain, sit in bath

Prescription
- topical fusidic acid for mild infections
- co-amoxiclav for 7 days if cellulitis (erythromycin if allergic to penicillin)

Refer to GP
- routinely:
  - adults, if severe symptoms or swab negative (may need referral to genitourinary clinic)
  - if recurrent episodes

Caution
- if no visible redness, this may be a UTI

- Schwartz RH (1996) Acute balanoposthitis in young boys. *Paed Inf Dis.* **15**(2): 176–7.

5 Gynaecology

Vaginal discharge

History
- duration
- colour
- smell
- itch
- abdominal pain
- fever
- irregular bleeding
- previous episodes
- timing with menstrual cycle

Examination
- not necessary if both you and the patient are sure it is due to candida (thrush)
- check for retained tampon
- look for 'cottage cheese' appearance of thrush

Tests
- high vaginal swab (HVS)
- consider cervical swabs for bacterial and chlamydial tests if diagnosis not obvious
- if recurrent thrush, test blood glucose

Action
- if thrush:
  - clotrimazole pessary
  - miconazole/hydrocortisone ointment
- if diagnosis uncertain wait for HVS result
- no need to treat partner unless he has symptoms

- if recurrent, suggest cotton pants, and avoid tights, bubble bath and biological washing powders

Refer to GP
- same day if:
  - abdominal pain
  - fever
  - genital blisters
- routinely if:
  - recurrent symptoms

Caution
- genital herpes – causes:
  - blisters
  - pain rather than itch
- pelvic inflammatory disease – causes:
  - abdominal pain
  - fever
  - irregular bleeding

- Woolley PD and Higgins SP (1995) Comparison of clotrimazole, fluconazole and itraconazole in vaginal candidiasis. *Br J Clin Pract.* **49**(2): 65–6.

Menorrhagia (heavy periods)

History
- duration of this period
- usual pattern of menstrual cycle
- clots/flooding
- previous episodes
- intrauterine contraceptive device (IUCD) fitted?
- was this period late?
- is it a possible miscarriage?
- any hot flushes/sweats (if aged over 40)?

Examination	• not necessary urgently
Tests	• consider FBC/thyroid function test (TFT) if recurrent problem
	• and follicle-stimulating hormone (FSH) on day 10 of cycle if menopause suspected
Action	• reassure patient there is no link between 'clots' and 'thrombosis'
	• ferrous sulphate
	• ibuprofen or tranexamic acid } until bleeding stops
	• if the above fail, norethisterone for 10 days will stop the bleeding. A light period will occur after stopping tablets
Refer to GP	• for vaginal examination/smear once bleeding has stopped
Caution	• miscarriage

Missed pills

History	• how far into this packet?
	• how many missed pills?
	• how late?
	• type of pill: combined or progestogen-only
Examination	• none
Tests	• none
Action	• advise the patient to take the last missed pill now, then resume normal pill-taking, **but**
	• **if combined oral contraceptive:**
	– if two or more pills have been missed from the first seven in the COC pack and intercourse has occurred since the end of the last pack, consider emergency contraception (*see* pages 73–4)

- if 12 or more hours late, contraceptive protection will be lost; continue the pill and, for the next 7 days, use a condom also, or refrain from intercourse

- if these 7 days run beyond the end of the packet, do not have a gap: start the next packet immediately; in this situation, patient may not have a period, or may have unexpected bleeding

- **if progestogen-only contraceptive:**

   - if 3 or more hours late and intercourse has occurred since the last pill was taken, consider emergency contraception (*see* pages 73–4)

   - if 3 or more hours late, contraceptive protection will be lost. For the next 48 h use a condom also, or refrain from intercourse

- check GMS4 form is current

- Guillebaud J (1998) *Contraception Today*. Martin Dunitz, London.

Intermenstrual bleeding

History
- menstrual cycle/date of last menstrual period (LMP)
- previous episodes
- fever
- abdominal pain
- offensive discharge
- any possibility of pregnancy?
- oral contraceptive?
   - missed pills/vomiting/antibiotic
- contraceptive method
- taking hormone replacement therapy (HRT)

Examination
- not necessary unless pain/fever/discharge present, in which case refer

Tests	• consider pregnancy test
Action	• make appointment for smear, when bleeding stops, if no smear in last 12 months
	• if missed pills/vomiting/antibiotic:
	– *see* missed pill advice (page 71)
	• if unexplained bleeding on oral or injectable contraceptive, make routine family planning appointment
Refer to GP	• immediately if abdominal pain/fever/offensive discharge (could be pelvic inflammatory disease)/pregnant
	• routinely if on oral or injectable contraceptive, HRT or no obvious cause for symptom
Caution	• very rarely, carcinoma of cervix/uterus/ovary may present in this way

Emergency oral contraception

History	• date of LMP
	• time since unprotected sexual intercourse (must be 72 h or less)
	• previous unprotected sexual intercourse this cycle (may render treatment ineffective – consider IUCD)
Examination	• check blood pressure if not measured in last 6 months
Tests	• none
Action	• give leaflet and advice:
	– may cause nausea
	– seek help if vomits within 2 h of taking tablet
	– use barrier method until next period, which may be early or late
	– only 0.4% failure rate if taken within 24 h of intercourse

– advise pregnancy test if next period more than 1 week late

– no known adverse effect on foetus if pregnancy occurs

– discuss long-term contraception

– complete GMS4 form, if not current

Prescription
- two levonorgestrel 750 µg tablets, one to be taken as soon as possible, but consider timing in order to avoid having to set alarm clock for second dose. The other tablet is taken 12 h later

Refer to GP
- if more than 72 h since unprotected intercourse
- if pregnant

Caution
- if patient vomits within 2 h of taking either dose, give replacement prescription for two tablets, also domperidone tablets to be taken 30 minutes before levonorgestrel dose

- WHO (1998) Randomised controlled trial of levonorgestrel versus the Yuzpe regime of combined oral contraceptives for emergency contraception. *Lancet.* **352**: 428–33.

Emergency IUCD contraception

History
- LMP
- past history of:
  - pelvic inflammatory disease
  - ectopic pregnancy
  - operations on fallopian tubes

Examination
- will be done by clinician fitting IUCD

Tests
- cervical swab for chlamydia

Action
- an IUCD can be fitted up to day 19 of a 28-day cycle, regardless of the date of unprotected intercourse; the factors listed above are contraindications

- give leaflet
- book appointment
- complete GMS4 form

Mastitis (in a breastfeeding woman)

History	• fever
	• pain
	• redness of breast
Examination	• record area of redness
	• any suggestion of an abscess?
Tests	• none
Action	• advise continue breastfeeding (unless pus from nipple)
	• offer affected breast to baby first, to ensure good drainage
Prescription	• flucloxacillin for 7 days (erythromycin if the patient is allergic to penicillin)
Refer to GP	• if abscess formation

6 Mental health

Depression

History
- how long has the patient felt low?
- any special reason, e.g. bereavement, post-partum, relationship difficulties, financial worries, stress at work?
- previous episodes and treatment
- medication
- sleep disturbance
- appetite or weight change
- suicidal thoughts: 'have you ever felt that life wasn't worth living?'
- loss of concentration
- poor memory
- lack of enthusiasm/enjoyment: 'what are you looking forward to?'
- alcohol intake
- street drugs

Examination
- none

Tests
- none

Action
- empathise
- if taking regular medication, check listed side effects in the *British National Formulary* (*BNF*)
- discuss referral to counsellor, or other form of talking therapy
- discuss antidepressants – emphasise not addictive/ effective/3 week delay before onset of action/course will last several months
- St John's wort is effective in treating mild depression

Refer to GP
- may be urgent, if symptoms are severe or suicidal thoughts are expressed

Caution
- some drugs can cause depression

- St John's wort interacts with: combined oral contraceptives/ triptan drugs (for migraine)/SSRI anti-depressants/anti-convulsants/warfarin/digoxin/theophylline/cyclosporin/ anti-viral drugs used in HIV infection

- Linde K, Ramirez G, Mulrow C *et al.* (1996) St John's wort for depression: an overview and meta-analysis of randomised clinical trials. *BMJ.* **313**: 253–8.

Insomnia

Insomnia is common and subjective. Some people only require 4 or 5 hours sleep a night, whereas others need 10 hours or more. The amount of sleep required tends to lessen with age and also with lower activity levels. A 'good' night's sleep is not the same for everyone. Almost everyone will have periods of insomnia at some stage.

History
- what is the patient's concern about the sleeping pattern?
- when did the problem start?
- what is the sleep pattern?
  - difficulty getting off to sleep
  - recurrent waking during the night
  - early morning waking feeling unrefreshed
- what was pattern like previously?
- what are the patient's expectations? – explore their ideas
- does the patient take daytime naps?
- does their partner say that they snore and are restless?

Consider causes:

- physical: pain, itching, shortness of breath, nocturia, indigestion, tinnitus, discomfort, too warm, too cold, noise, room not dark

- physiological: shift work, jet lag, pregnancy

- psychological: depression, emotional upsets, worries, bereavement, hypomania

- psychiatric: especially depression

- pharmacological: is patient on any medication possibly causing insomnia, e.g. corticosteroids, propranolol, pseudoephedrine, or taking coffee, tea, cola, alcohol, cigarettes in evening, or excessive laxatives

- social: new baby, enuretic child, partner who has nocturia or who snores

Examination
- look for agitation, depression, 'washed out' appearance

Tests
- none

Action
- deal with underlying cause

Advice
- avoid going to bed until you feel sleepy

- take a warm, milky drink before bedtime

- regular exercise is helpful, but not just before bedtime

- relaxation exercises can be helpful; also yoga, t'ai chi, meditation, reading and listening to soft music

- avoid lying in bed unable to get to sleep – it is better to get up and do something you do not enjoy, e.g. ironing

- try to wake at the same time each day using an alarm clock and do not sleep on

- hypnotic drugs such as temazepam may cause tolerance, addiction, daytime drowsiness and rebound insomnia on stopping. It is therefore best to avoid these drugs. If essential, give temazepam 10 mg tablets one at night for a maximum of 5 days

Refer to GP
- if psychiatric problem

- if problem is due to prescribed drugs or treatable physical cause

- if obese and reporting snoring and excessive tiredness (may need assessment for sleep apnoea syndrome)

Anxiety/panic/phobias

History
- active, sympathetic listening
- why have they come?
- problems at work? at home? relatives? financial?
- alcohol intake
- street drugs
- previous problems

Examination
- none

Tests
- take blood for TFTs if not recently done

Action
- empathise
- ask 'how can the practice help?'
- consider practical suggestions
  - suggest useful books (*see* Recommended reading)
  - referral agencies:
    - (i)   counsellor (or other talking therapy)
    - (ii) health visitor
    - (iii) community psychiatric nurse
    - (iv) Citizens Advice service
    - (v) Samaritans
  - would time off work help?
  - consider relaxation techniques/yoga/t'ai chi/meditation

Refer to GP
- if drug treatment requested or follow-up required

Hyperventilation

History
- 'unable to take a deep breath'
- no cough/malaise

- precipitating stress
- previous episodes
- tingling round mouth, hands, feet
- spasm of hands and feet (tetany)

$\rightarrow\rightarrow\rightarrow\rightarrow\rightarrow\rightarrow\rightarrow$ **anxiety** $\rightarrow\rightarrow\rightarrow\rightarrow\rightarrow\rightarrow\rightarrow\rightarrow$

↑   ↓
↑   ↓

strange feelings,   faster breathing
tingling, faintness   ↓

↑   ↓
↑   ↓
$\leftarrow\leftarrow\leftarrow\leftarrow\leftarrow\leftarrow$ reduction in $\leftarrow\leftarrow\leftarrow\leftarrow\leftarrow\leftarrow$
blood carbon dioxide

Examination
- respiratory rate – irregular or sighing?
- listen to chest – absent breath sounds on one side? (pneumothorax)
- wheeze? (asthma)
- record peak flow (if low, *see* asthma)

Action
- explain problem
- get patient to breathe slowly in and out of paper bag

Refer to GP
- urgently if:
  - unequal/abnormal breath sounds
  - peak flow less than 75% of predicted value
  - problem does not respond promptly to treatment
- routinely if:
  - underlying stresses need attention
  - breathing pattern remains disturbed (may need physio-therapy referral)

7 Injuries

Minor injuries

History
- severity of impact (may suggest likely consequences)
- impairment of function

Examination
- swelling
- deformity
- restriction of movement

Action
- **m**obilise

MINE
- **i**ce (e.g. pack of frozen peas, wrapped in a towel to avoid skin damage)
- **N**SAID if tolerated, e.g. ibuprofen
- **e**levation

(Compression is a traditional treatment which is no longer recommended)

- Wilson S and Cooke M (1998) Double bandaging of sprained ankles. *BMJ.* **317**: 1722–3.

Refer to A&E if
- deformity
- severe pain
- bony tenderness
- unable to bear weight on leg

Road traffic accident – assessment

History
- date and time of the accident
- details of the accident

- if in a car, whether a seat belt was worn and whether there was a head restraint; whether passenger or driver

- what are the patient's descriptions of the injuries: pain, stiffness, bruising, etc?

- psychological effects: shaking, insomnia, nightmares, fear of driving, flashbacks

- time off work

Examination
- appropriate to affected area

- extent of grazing and bruising – measure these – diagram may help

- movement of affected limbs or neck

Tests
- none (usually)

Action
- give treatment and advice dependent on and appropriate to the injuries

- advise patient to photograph grazing and bruising

Caution
- often the main purpose of the patient's visit is to document the injuries for a possible future compensation claim. Record the details carefully

8 Certificates

NHS certificates

These are not issued for periods of less than a week: the patient should obtain an SC2 form from his or her employer, or an SC1 from the surgery if self-employed or unemployed.

Certificates can be backdated if the patient has previously been seen by a GP, deputising service doctor or hospital doctor (pink form: MED 5). No certificate can be forward dated.

Closed certificates (with a return-to-work date) can only be given if the date is within 14 days of the date of issue.

In some areas the Benefits Agency has agreed that a named nurse with a minor illness qualification may sign certificates.

Private certificates

These can be issued at the recommended British Medical Association (BMA) rate, which should be reclaimed from the employer.

9 Notifiable diseases

Diseases which must be notified to the Consultant in Communicable Disease Control (CCDC) on the appropriate form include:

- food poisoning
- suspected food poisoning
- measles
- mumps
- rubella
- pertussis.

A full list is given on the cover of the book of notification forms.

Warn the patient that he or she may be contacted by a doctor from the Public Health Department.

If there are any implications for the community, e.g. suspected food poisoning in a chef or a rare infectious disease, notify the local consultant in communicable disease by telephone or fax.

Table 9.1.   Exclusion and infectiousness

Disease	Incubation period	Infective period	Exclude from school	
			Case	Home contact
Chickenpox	2–3 weeks	From 1 day before until 6 days after rash appears	6 days from onset of rash	None
Conjunctivitis	1–3 days	While discharge present	Until discharge stops	None
Food poisoning	1–3 days	While diarrhoea lasts	Until well and no diarrhoea	None unless bacteria found, when CCDC* will decide
Glandular fever	33–49 days	While symptomatic	Until well	None
Hand, foot and mouth disease	3–5 days	As long as active ulcers are present	1 week or until lesions healed	None
Head lice	7–10 days	As long as lice or live eggs are present	Until child and family have been treated	None
Impetigo	1–3 days	While purulent lesions persist	Until skin has healed, or 48 h after treatment started	None
Parvovirus (slapped cheek)	4–14 days	Until rash appears	None	None
Scabies	2–6 days	Until mites and eggs have been destroyed	Until day after treatment	None once treated
Threadworms	2–6 weeks	As long as eggs present on perianal skin	None once treated	None once treated
Tinea of head or body	1–2 weeks	While lesions are active	Only if epidemic suspected	None
Tinea of feet (athlete's foot)	Unknown	While lesions are active	Only if epidemic suspected	None
Tonsillitis or streptococcal throat infection	1–3 days	Up to 48 h after antibiotic	Until better (usually 48 h after antibiotic)	None
Verrucae (plantar warts)	4 months	As long as wart present	None (cover wart with waterproof dressing for swimming/barefoot sports)	None
Whooping cough	1–3 weeks	1 week before until 3 weeks after onset of cough	3 weeks	None

Based on guidelines from Bedfordshire Health (1993).
*Consultant in Communicable Disease Control.

10 Suggested specialist nurses' formulary

Notes on prescribing

Some practices will already have a practice or district formulary, e.g. Bedfordshire Primary Care Formulary www.wlhc.demon.co.uk/formulary/index.htm. Most of the drugs listed here are 'basic' and will probably be included in local formularies also, but it may be wise to cross-check.

Drugs marked 'OTC' are available over the counter, and often cost less than a prescription charge. The price depends on the pack size, brand and pharmacy.

Under current regulations, prescriptions must still be signed by a doctor; but if the nurse can complete the details of the prescription and slip it under the doctor's door for signature, the interruption will be minimal. The only exception to this is a qualified Nurse Prescriber, who can prescribe from the limited list of items in the *Nurse Prescribing Formulary*.

The FP10 prescription pad has a box at the top where the number of days' treatment may be entered. This reduces the need to calculate quantities but cannot be used for 'as required' drugs, creams, lotions, etc.

The following are brief notes: the *British National Formulary* and its appendices should be consulted for full information. Always check for interaction with any other current medication, allergy, pregnancy and breast-feeding. Some drugs are contraindicated, or should be given at lower dosage, in patients with kidney, liver or heart failure. If in doubt, consult the doctor.

Previous antibiotic treatment

If a patient presents with a condition requiring antibiotic treatment, but has finished a course of the 'first-choice' antibiotic within the last 7 days, then either the infection is viral or the organism is resistant to the antibiotic. In these circumstances a different antibiotic may be necessary, as follows:

- for otitis media or sinusitis – change to co-amoxiclav
- for chest infections – add erythromycin or change to doxycycline (*see* notes on mycoplasma infection, page 11)

- for throat infections – take throat swab and await result before prescribing a different antibiotic, as in most cases the infection will be viral.

Antibiotics and oral contraceptives

Broad-spectrum antibiotics may slightly reduce the effectiveness of the combined oral contraceptive pill. Advise patients to use a condom or refrain from intercourse while taking the antibiotic and for 1 week afterwards.

Narrow-spectrum antibiotics such as penicillin V, flucloxacillin and trimethoprim do not have this effect.

The progestogen-only pill (minipill) is not affected by any of the antibiotics in this formulary.

Allergies

Many reported allergies are really just coincidences, for example, the appearance of a viral rash just after starting a course of antibiotic. However, any report of swelling of the tongue or face, or difficulty in breathing, must be taken seriously.

If the patient has a true allergy to one type of penicillin, *all* drugs of this class should be avoided. This does not apply if the patient experiences non-allergic side effects, such as diarrhoea with co-amoxiclav; penicillin V will probably not produce this side effect.

Ten percent of those allergic to penicillin will also be allergic to cefalexin.

▼ Black triangle symbol

This symbol means that there is limited experience of the use of this product and the Committee on Safety of Medicine (CSM) requests that *all* suspected adverse reactions should be reported. Use the yellow forms in the *BNF*.

Formulary

Formulary listed by *BNF* classification.

Gastrointestinal system

Magnesium trisilicate [1.1]
Cimetidine [1.3.1]
Loperamide [1.4.2]
Senna [1.6.2]
Lactulose [1.6.4]
Anusol® [1.7.1]
Xyloproct® [1.7.2]

Cardiovascular system

Tranexamic acid [2.11]

Respiratory system

Salbutamol [3.1]
Terbutaline [3.1]
Volumatic [3.1.4]
Peak flow meter [3.1.5]
Beclometasone inhaler [3.2]
Fexofenadine [3.4.1]
Loratadine [3.4.1]
Chlorpheniramine [3.4.1]
Menthol and Eucalyptus [3.8]
Pholcodine [3.9]
Pseudoephedrine [3.10]

Nervous system

Temazepam [4.1.1]
Prochlorperazine [4.6]
Domperidone [4.6]
Aspirin [4.7.1]
Paracetamol [4.7.1]
Co-codamol 30/500 [4.7.1]
Codeine phosphate [4.7.2]
Dihydrocodeine [4.7.2]

Infection

Penicillin V [5.1.1]
Flucloxacillin [5.1.1.2]
Amoxicillin [5.1.1.3]
Co-amoxiclav [5.1.1.3]
Cefalexin [5.1.2]
Doxycycline [5.1.3]
Erythromycin [5.1.5]
Clarithromycin [5.1.5]
Trimethoprim [5.1.8]
Metronidazole [5.1.11]
Nitrofurantoin MR [5.1.13]
Nystatin [5.2]
Mebendazole [5.5.1]
Piperazine [5.5.1]

Endocrine system

Norethisterone [6.4.1.2]

Obstetrics and gynaecology

Clotrimazole [7.2.2]
Levonorgestrel [7.3.1]

Nutrition and blood

Ferrous sulphate [9.1.1]
Dioralyte® [9.2.1.2]

Musculoskeletal system

Ibuprofen [10.1.1]
Intralgin® [10.3.2]

Eye

Chloramphenicol [11.3.1]
Sodium cromoglicate [11.4.2]
Hypromellose [11.8.1]

Ear, nose and oropharynx

Otosporin® [12.1.1]
Beclometasone aqueous spray [12.2.1]
Saline nose drops [12.2.2]
Steam inhalation [12.2.2]
Adcortyl in Orabase® [12.3.1]

Skin

Emulsifying ointment [13.2.1]
Hydrous ointment [13.2.1]
Sudocrem® [13.2.1]
Oilatum® [13.2.1.1]
Hydrocortisone [13.4]
Eumovate® [13.4]
Betnovate® [13.4]
Miconazole/Hydrocortisone [13.4]
Glutaraldehyde [13.7]
Fusidic acid [13.10.1]
Aciclovir [13.10.3]
Malathion [13.10.4]
Lyclear [13.10.4]

Gastrointestinal system

[1.1] Magnesium trisilicate (OTC)

Oral suspension:	magnesium trisilicate, light magnesium carbonate, sodium bicarbonate, peppermint flavour
Tablets:	magnesium trisilicate 250 mg, aluminium hydroxide 120 mg
Dose:	10 ml suspension three times daily in water *or* 1–2 tablets chewed when required
Side effects:	the suspension may cause diarrhoea occasionally
Interactions:	may reduce the absorption of some other drugs **w**arfarin, **i**ron, **N**SAID, **d**igoxin ('*wind*')
Cautions:	as the mixture contains sodium (equivalent to about 3 level teaspoonfuls of salt in a 500 ml bottle), it should be used with caution when there is heart failure, hypertension, renal or hepatic failure

[1.3.1] Cimetidine (lower dose tablets available OTC)

Tablets:	400, 800 mg
Dose:	400 mg twice daily *or* 800 mg at night
Side effects:	all of these are **rare**, cimetidine is usually well tolerated: altered bowel habit, dizziness, rash, tiredness, confusion, headache; very rarely, liver or kidney damage, muscle or joint pain, bradycardia and heart block, acute pancreatitis, blood disorders; impotence and breast tissue enlargement are also occasional problems with cimetidine but usually only in high dosage
Interactions:	there are many interactions, so always check any other medication in Appendix 1 of the *BNF*. Some important ones: cimetidine inhibits the enzymes which deactivate: warfarin, phenytoin (Epanutin®), propranolol and theophylline
Cautions:	liver and kidney disease pregnancy and breastfeeding

[1.4.2] Loperamide (OTC)

Capsules:	2 mg
Dose:	two capsules initially, followed by one after each loose stool for up to a maximum of 5 days; usual dose 3–4 capsules a day, maximum of 8 capsules a day

[1.6.2] Glycerol suppositories (OTC)

Suppositories:	1, 2, 4 g (box of 12) gelatin 140 mg, glycerol 700 mg, purified water to 1 g

Dose:	adults	4 g	one inserted into rectum
	children	2 g	as required
	infants	1 g	moisten with water before use

[1.6.2] Senna (OTC)

Tablets:	7.5 mg
Syrup:	7.5 mg/5 ml

Dose: adults   15–30 mg at night
children   2–6 years: 3.75–7.5 mg at night
6–12 years: 7.5–15 mg at night

Side effect: abdominal cramp

Cautions: bowel obstruction
prolonged use can cause an atonic,
non-functioning colon and hypokalaemia

[1.6.4] Lactulose (OTC)

Solution: 3.3 g/5 ml in pack of 200 ml

Powder: 10 g sachet (equivalent to 15 ml of solution)

Dose: *These are suggested starting doses, which may need adjustment according to response.*
adults   15 ml twice a day
children   under 1 year: 2.5 ml twice a day
1–5 years: 5 ml twice a day
5–10 years: 10 ml twice a day

Side effect: flatulence

Caution: intestinal obstruction, galactosaemia

[1.7.1] Anusol® (OTC)

Ointment: 25 g

Suppositories: 12 or 24 in a pack

Dose: one suppository inserted   } night and morning
or one application of ointment } and after defecation

[1.7.2] Xyloproct®

Ointment: 30 g

Suppositories: 10 in a pack

Dose: one suppository inserted at night and after a bowel movement or application of ointment several times a day

Side effect: dermatitis

Cautions: pregnancy, anal infections such as *herpes simplex* or candida

Cardiovascular system

[2.1.1] Tranexamic acid

Tablets:	500 mg
Dose:	adults: 1–3 tablets up to four times a day
Side effects:	**rare**: nausea, vomiting, diarrhoea (reduce dose)
Cautions:	previous thrombosis
	reduce dose in renal disease

Respiratory system

[3.1.1] Salbutamol CFC-free and Ventolin Easi-Breathe® inhaler

Inhaler:	100 µg per dose
Nebuliser solution:	2.5 mg/2.5 ml, 5 mg/2.5 ml

Dose: inhaler: child 1–2 doses four times a day if required
                           adult 2 doses four times a day if required
         nebulised: child 2.5 mg four times a day
                           adult 5 mg four times a day

Side effects: fine tremor (usually hands), nervous tension, headache, tachycardia, hypokalaemia

Interactions: high doses of salbutamol can cause dangerous hypokalaemia, particularly in combination with corticosteroids, diuretics or theophylline

Cautions: hyperthyroidism, ischaemic heart disease, hypertension, any pedisposing factors to hypokalaemia

[3.1.1] Terbutaline

Syrup:	1.5 mg/5 ml in 300 ml pack
Dose:	child: 0.25 ml of syrup/kg three times a day
Side effects:	tremor, sleep and behavioural disturbance, hypokalaemia
Interactions:	greater risk of hypokalaemia in combination with corticosteroids, diuretics or theophylline

[3.1.4] Volumatic® (OTC)

spacer device with or without paediatric mask

[3.1.5] Peak flow meter

Device: standard range for adults, low range for children

[3.2] Beclometasone inhaler and Becotide Easi-Breathe®

Inhaler: 50, 100 and 200 µg per dose

Dose: *see* text on acute asthma, 100–800 µg/day

Side effects: may precipitate oral thrush
                wash mouth out after use
                use spacer if high doses needed
                rarely: glaucoma, cataracts

Caution: active or quiescent tuberculosis

[3.4.1] Fexofenadine ▼

Tablets: 120, 180 mg

Dose: adults   120–180 mg once a day
                children over 12 years 120 mg once a day

Side effects: incidence of sedation is low but it is still worth
                warning drivers to be alert to the slight possibility of
                drowsiness or dizziness

Cautions: pregnancy, prostatic hypertrophy, urinary retention,
                glaucoma, hepatic disease, epilepsy, porphyria

[3.4.1] Loratadine (OTC)

Tablets:	10 mg
Syrup:	5 mg/5 ml
Dose:	adults: 10 mg daily children over 30 kg weight: 10 mg daily children under 30 kg weight: 5 mg daily
Side effects:	incidence of sedation is low; rarely: fatigue, nausea and headache
Cautions:	prostatic hypertrophy, urinary retention, glaucoma, hepatic disease, epilepsy, porphyria

[3.4.1] Chlorpheniramine (OTC)

Tablets:	4 mg
Elixir:	2 mg/5 ml

Dose:	adults 4 mg every 4–6 h, max 24 mg daily
	children 1–2 years: 1 mg twice a day
	         2–5 years: 1 mg every 4–6 h, max 6 mg daily
	         6–12 years: 1 mg every 4–6 h, max 12 mg daily

Side effects:	drowsiness may affect performance of skilled tasks, e.g. driving; headache, psychomotor impairment, dry mouth, blurred vision and gastrointestinal disturbances, rashes, photosensitivity and paradoxical stimulation
Cautions:	prostatic hypertrophy, urinary retention, glaucoma, hepatic disease, epilepsy, porphyria
Interactions:	tricyclic antidepressants, sedatives

[3.8] Menthol & Eucalyptus (OTC)

Dose: add one teaspoonful to a pint of hot water and inhale vapour

Side effect: only burns from spilling the water

Cautions: use hot, not boiling, water
                 may induce apnoea in infants less than 3 months

[3.9] Pholcodine (OTC)

Linctus: 2 mg/5 ml, 5 mg/5 ml, 10 mg/5 ml (sugar-free versions available)

Dose: all three times a day
                 adults   5–10 mg
                 children   1–5 years   2 mg
                             5–12 years   2.5–5 mg

Side effects: constipation, in large doses respiratory depression

Interactions: mexiletine, monoamine oxidase inhibitor (MAOI) antidepressants, anxiolytics and hypnotics

Cautions: asthma, hepatic and renal impairment, history of drug abuse

[3.10] Pseudoephedrine (OTC)

Tablets: 60, 120 mg

Elixir: 30 mg/5 ml

Dose: all three times a day
                 adults   60 mg
                 children   2–6 years   15 mg
                             6–12 years   30 mg

Side effects: insomnia if taken in the evening, anxiety

Interactions: **MAOI antidepressants**

Cautions: hypertension, hyperthyroidism, coronary heart disease, diabetes mellitus. Can affect judgement, therefore banned by Civil Aviation Authority for use by pilots or air traffic controllers on duty

Nervous system

[4.1.1] Temazepam

Tablets:	10 mg
Dose:	one at night, maximum supply: 5 tablets
Side effects:	drowsiness and lightheadedness the next day; confusion and ataxia (especially in the elderly); tolerance on long-term use
Interactions:	enhanced sedation with: **cisapride**, alcohol, opiates, tricyclic antidepressants, antihistamines, antipsychotics, disulfram, lofexidine, baclofen, tizanidine, cimetidine
Cautions:	potentially addictive, may cause daytime drowsiness, increases the effect of alcohol. Do not use in those with chronic chest disease, liver or renal disease, or in pregnancy or breastfeeding. May affect driving the following day

[4.6] Prochlorperazine

Tablets: 5 mg

Buccal tablets: 3 mg

Syrup: 5 mg/5 ml

Suppositories: 5, 25 mg

Dose: adults only
                  tablets/syrup   5 mg three times a day for labyrinthine
                                  disorders
                  higher doses may be needed for nausea and vomiting
                  – see BNF

Buccal tablets: 1 or 2 tablets twice a day
                  place high between lip and gum and leave to dissolve

Suppositories: 25 mg inserted into rectum followed by oral dose
                  after 6 h or for migraine, 5 mg suppository three times
                  a day

Side effects: for a full list see the BNF under chlorpromazine, but
                  in practice the only common one is drowsiness, and
                  very occasionally severe dystonic reactions (see
                  below)

Interactions: desferrioxamine, dopaminergic drugs in Parkinson's
                  disease, lithium

Cautions: may cause severe dystonic reactions (abnormal face
                  and body movements). This is rare, but more
                  common in teenagers and the very elderly. Best to
                  avoid in these age groups

[4.6] **Domperidone** (OTC)

Tablets:	10 mg
Suspension:	5 mg/5 ml
Suppositories:	30 mg

Dose:
adults only
oral   10–20 mg every 4–8 h
rectal   30–60 mg every 4–8 h

Side effects: raised prolactin concentrations (possible breast tissue enlargement and leakage of milk from the nipples); reduced libido and acute dystonic reactions reported (*see* under prochlorperazine)

Cautions: renal impairment, pregnancy, breastfeeding
max duration of treatment 12 weeks

[4.7.1] **Aspirin** (OTC)

Tablets: 75 mg, 300 mg (dispersible also available)

Dose and indications:
adult doses, ideally taken with or after food
anti-thrombotic use   75–300 mg daily
analgesic use (rarely the
   best drug for this)   600 mg four times a day
after by-pass surgery   75–100 mg daily
after myocardial infarction 150 mg daily
transient ischaemic attack   300 mg daily
Not for use by children under 12

Side effects: high incidence of gastrointestinal irritation with slight asymptomatic blood loss, increased bleeding time, bronchospasm and skin reactions in hypersensitive patients

Cautions: allergy, peptic ulcer, pregnancy, breastfeeding, interaction with warfarin, asthma (a small proportion of asthmatic patients find that aspirin worsens their symptoms; occasionally this can be severe)

[4.7.1] Paracetamol (OTC)

Tablets:	500 mg
Soluble tablets:	500 mg
Paediatric sol tablets:	120 mg
Suspension:	250 mg/5 ml, 120 mg/5 ml
Suppositories:	60, 125, 250, 500 mg

Dose: all four times a day
adults   500–1000 mg
children 3 months–1 year   60–120 mg
1–5 years   120–250 mg
6–12 years   250–500 mg

Side effect: overdose is the only serious problem

Interactions: possibly enhances warfarin, cholestyramine reduces absorption of paracetamol, metoclopramide accelerates it

Caution: overdosage with paracetamol is particularly dangerous as it may cause hepatic damage which is sometimes not apparent for 4 to 6 days

[4.7.1] Co-codamol 30/500

Tablets, effervescent tablets and capsules
containing codeine phosphate 30 mg and paracetamol 500 mg

Dose: adults only
1–2 tablets 4-hourly as required,
maximum 8 in 24 h

Side effects: overdose, constipation, may cause drowsiness

Caution: overdosage with paracetamol is particularly dangerous as it may cause hepatic damage which is sometimes not apparent for 4 to 6 days

[4.7.2] Codeine phosphate

Tablets:	30 mg
Dose:	adults only 1 tablet 4-hourly as required
Side effects:	constipation, nausea, dependence, may cause drowsiness
Interactions:	alcohol, sedatives, MAOI antidepressants, selegiline
Caution:	to take this drug abroad, patients may require a letter from their doctor stating that it is a necessary medication

[4.7.2] Dihydrocodeine

Tablets:	30 mg
Dose:	adults only 30 mg four times a day
Side effects:	nausea, constipation, drowsiness, dependence, vertigo
Interactions:	alcohol, sedatives, MAOI antidepressants, selegiline
Cautions:	respiratory disease, liver or renal failure, hypothyroidism, pregnancy (3rd trimester)

Infection

[5.1.1] Penicillin V

Tablets: 250 mg

Oral suspension: 125 mg/5 ml, 250 mg/5 ml

Dose: all four times a day
                             adults   500 mg, increased to 750 mg in severe
                                          infections
                             children   up to 1 year   62.5 mg
                                         1–5 years   125 mg
                                         6–12 years   250 mg

Side effects: hypersensitivity reactions including urticaria,
                             fever, joint pains, rashes, angioedema,
                             anaphylaxis, haemolytic anaemia and interstitial
                             nephritis

Interactions: penicillin V is not a broad-spectrum antibiotic and
                             therefore does not affect the combined oral
                             contraceptive or warfarin

Caution: penicillin allergy

[5.1.1.2] Flucloxacillin

Capsules:	250, 500 mg
Oral solution:	125 mg/5 ml, 250 mg/5 ml
Dose:	all four times a day, at least 30 minutes before food
	doses may be doubled in severe infection

adults and children over 10   250 mg
children   up to 2 years   62.5 mg
           2–10 years   125 mg

Side effects:	*see* penicillin V; rare: hepatitis, cholestatic jaundice
Interactions:	flucloxacillin is a narrow-spectrum antibiotic and therefore does not affect the combined oral contraceptive or warfarin
Cautions:	penicillin allergy, porphyria
	syrup tastes awful, children may not like the taste; co-amoxiclav is an alternative, though broader spectrum

[5.1.1.3] Amoxicillin

Capsules:	250, 500 mg
Oral suspension:	125 mg/5 ml, 250 mg/5 ml
Drops:	125 mg/1.25 ml (20 ml bottle)
Dose:	adults and children over 10: 250 mg three times a day children up to 10 years: 125 mg three times a day doses for any age group can be doubled in severe infections
Side effects:	nausea, diarrhoea, rashes, allergic reactions
Interactions:	warfarin effect may be altered, slight reduction in efficacy of combined oral contraceptive pill
Caution:	allergy

[5.1.1.3] Co-amoxiclav

A mixture of amoxicillin and clavulanic acid

Oral suspension:	400/57 mg in 5 ml: 35, 70 ml bottle
Tablet:	250/125 mg (= 375) or 500/125 mg (= 625)
Dose:	adults: 375 mg three times a day
	increased to 625 mg in severe infections
	children **using 400/57 mg suspension**:
	(be careful to specify the strength of the
	suspension as there are several types)
	2 months–2 years: 0.15 ml *per kg* twice a day
	2–6 years 2.5 ml twice a day
	7–12 years 5 ml twice a day
Side effects:	nausea, diarrhoea, rashes, hepatitis
	cholestatic jaundice: 1 in 6000 risk of liver
	damage (greater in elderly/rare in children)
Interactions:	warfarin effect may be altered, slight reduction in
	efficacy of combined oral contraceptive pill
Caution:	penicillin allergy

[5.1.2] Cefalexin

Tablets or capsules:	250, 500 mg
Oral suspension:	125 mg/5 ml, 250 mg/5 ml

Dose:

adults:	250 mg four times a day, or 500 mg two to three times a day	
children:	under 1 year	125 mg twice a day
	1–5 years	125 mg three times a day
	6–12 years	250 mg three times a day

Side effects:

diarrhoea and rarely pseudomembranous colitis (CSM has warned both more likely with higher doses), nausea and vomiting; allergic reactions including rashes, pruritus, urticaria, serum sickness-like reactions with rashes, fever and arthralgia, and anaphylaxis; erythema multiforme, toxic epidermal necrolysis reported; eosinophilia rarely thrombocytopenia or neutropenia; disturbances in liver enzymes, transient hepatitis and cholestatic jaundice

other side effects reported include reversible interstitial nephritis, hyperactivity, nervousness, sleep disturbances, confusion, hypertonia and dizziness

Interactions:

warfarin effect may be altered, slight reduction in efficacy of combined oral contraceptive pill

Cautions:

penicillin sensitivity, renal impairment, porphyria

[5.1.3] Doxycycline

Capsules:	100 mg
Disp tablets:	100 mg
Dose:	adults 200 mg on first day, then 100 mg daily capsules should be swallowed whole with plenty of fluid during meals, while sitting or standing
Side effects:	photosensitivity (avoid exposure to sunlight or sunlamps) nausea, vomiting, diarrhoea; erythema (discontinue treatment); very rarely headache and visual disturbances may indicate benign intracranial hypertension; pseudomembranous colitis reported
Interactions:	antacids, anticoagulants, antiepileptics, calcium salts, iron, oral bismuth chelate (Pepto-Bismol® or De-Nol®)
Cautions:	pregnancy, breastfeeding, systemic lupus erythematosus (SLE), hepatic impairment, porphyria **Not for children under 12 years of age**

[5.1.5] Erythromycin

Enteric-coated tablets:	250, 500 mg
Oral suspension:	125 mg/5 ml, 250 mg/5 ml
Dose:	all four times a day adults and children 8 years or older: 250–500 mg children: up to 2 years 125 mg 2–8 years 250 mg
Side effects:	nausea, vomiting, abdominal discomfort, diarrhoea after large doses; reversible hearing loss also reported after large doses; if given for more than 14 days may occasionally cause cholestatic jaundice
Interactions:	amiodarone, **astemizole*** (*Hismanal*), bromocriptine, cabergoline, carbamazepine, **cimetidine** (*Tagamet*), **cisapride**, clozapine, ciclosporin, digoxin, disopyramide, ergotamine, midazolam, pimozide, sertindole, **terfenadine***, theophylline, warfarin, zopiclone
Contraindication:	porphyria
Cautions:	hepatic and renal impairment

* Although astemizole and terfenadine are no longer available, patients may have old supplies in their medicine cupboard.

[5.1.5] Clarithromycin

Tablets: 250, 500 mg

Oral suspension: 125 mg/5 ml

Granules: 250 mg/sachet

Dose:
all twice a day
adults: 250–500 mg
children: 8–11 kg (1–2 years) 62.5 mg (2.5 ml)
12–19 kg (3–6 years) 125 mg (5ml)
20–29 kg (7–9 years) 187.5 mg (7.5 ml)
30–40 kg (10–12 years) 250 mg (10 ml)

Side effects: may cause similar side effects to erythromycin; also headache, taste disturbances, stomatitis, glossitis, hepatitis, phlebitis

Interactions: amiodarone, **astemizole*** (*Hismanal*), bromocriptine, cabergoline, carbamazepine, **cimetidine** (*Tagamet*), **cisapride**, clozapine, ciclosporin, digoxin, disopyramide, ergotamine, midazolam, pimozide, sertindole, **terfenadine***, theophylline, warfarin, zopiclone

Contraindication: porphyria

Cautions: hepatic and renal impairment

* Although astemizole and terfenadine are no longer available, patients may have old supplies in their medicine cupboard.

[5.1.8] Trimethoprim

Tablets:	100 mg, 200 mg
Oral suspension:	50 mg/5 ml

Dose:

all twice a day

adults:	200 mg
children: 2–5 months	25 mg
6 months–5 years	50 mg
6–12 years	100 mg

Side effects:
blood and generalised skin disorders, especially in the elderly; gastrointestinal disturbances including nausea and vomiting, pruritus, rashes

Interactions:
anticoagulant effect of warfarin and antifolate effect of phenytoin possibly enhanced, antimalarial drugs containing pyrimethamine (Fansidar® and Maloprim®), ciclosporin, methotrexate. Does not affect the combined oral contraceptive pill

Cautions:
pregnancy, breastfeeding, renal impairment, porphyria, blood dyscrasias

[5.1.11] Metronidazole

Tablets:	200 mg

Dose:
200 mg three times a day for dental infections (different dosage regimens are used for other infections)

Side effects:
nausea (metallic taste in mouth), vomiting and gastrointestinal disturbances, rashes; rarely drowsiness, headache, dizziness, ataxia and darkening of urine

Interactions:
alcohol (interaction may cause facial flushing, throbbing headache, palpitations, nausea and vomiting), warfarin, cimetidine, lithium

Cautions:
alcoholism, liver disease

[5.1.13] Nitrofurantoin

Modified release capsules:	100 mg
Dose:	adults: one capsule twice a day with food
Side effects:	urine may be coloured yellow or brown, anorexia, nausea, (m/r versions less so) vomiting, diarrhoea, acute and chronic pulmonary reactions, peripheral neuropathy; also reported rash, pruritus, hepatitis, pancreatitis, arthralgia, blood disorders and transient alopecia
Interactions:	probenecid, magnesium trisilicate
Cautions:	avoid in renal failure, glucose-6-phosphate dehydrogenase (G6PD) deficiency or porphyria; caution in anaemia, diabetes mellitus, electrolyte imbalance, vitamin B and folate deficiency, hepatic impairment, susceptibiliity to peripheral neuropathy

[5.2] Nystatin

Oral suspension:	100 000 units/ml in a 30 ml bottle with pipette	
Dose:	child	1 ml four times a day
	newborn infant	1 ml once daily
Side effect:	oral irritation	

[5.5.1] Mebendazole (OTC tablets only)

Tablets (chewable): 100 mg

Oral suspension: 100 mg/5 ml

Dose: for threadworms
                     adults and children aged 2 years and older:
                     100 mg single dose (if re-infection occurs, a
                     second dose may be needed after 2–3 weeks)

Side effects: rarely abdominal pain, diarrhoea, allergic
                     reactions

Cautions: pregnancy (toxicity in *rats*), breastfeeding
                     Note: The package insert in the Vermox® pack
                     includes the statement that it is not suitable for
                     women known to be pregnant or children under
                     2 years

[5.5.1] Piperazine (OTC)

Elixir: 750 mg/5 ml as piperazine citrate

Dose: for threadworms
                     3 months–2 years: 0.3–0.5 ml/kg
                                         once daily for 7 days
                     repeated after 1 week if necessary
                     2 years or older: use mebendazole

Side effects: nausea, vomiting, colic, diarrhoea, allergic reactions

Cautions: liver or renal impairment, neurological disease
                     including epilepsy

Endocrine system

[6.4.1.2] Norethisterone

Tablets:	5 mg
Dose:	1 tablet three times a day for 10 days
Side effects:	acne, urticaria, fluid retention, weight changes, gut effects, change in libido, breast discomfort
Interaction:	ciclosporin
Cautions:	pregnancy, arterial disease, epilepsy, migraine

Obstetrics and gynaecology

[7.2.2] Clotrimazole (OTC)

Cream 1%:	20 g, 50 g
Pessaries:	500 mg
Combination pack:	contains one 500 mg pessary plus 20 g of 1% cream
Vaginal cream 10%:	5 g
Dose:	for vaginal thrush: one 500 mg pessary or 5 g of 10% vaginal cream inserted at night
Side effects:	possible effect on latex condoms and diaphragms

---

[7.3.1] Levonorgestrel

Pack:	2 tablets of levonorgestrel 750 µg
Dose:	1 tablet as soon as possible (and not later than 72 h) after unprotected intercourse, followed by a second tablet 12 h after the first
Side effects:	generally less likely than with Schering PC4®, nausea 25%, vomiting 5%. The timing of menstrual bleeding may be temporarily disturbed, although most women have their next period on time. If it is more than 1 week overdue, a pregnancy test is needed. Glucose tolerance may worsen *rarely*: breast tenderness, headache, dizziness and tiredness
Interactions:	some anticonvulsants, ampicillin and rifampicin
Cautions:	check that there was no earlier unprotected intercourse during the same cycle that would be outside the 72-h limit. Also check that a period is not overdue – she may be pregnant already. May cause vomiting – if vomiting occurs within 2 h of taking a tablet, repeat with anti-emetic (domperidone). Hypertension, diabetes, ischaemic heart disease, stroke or history of breast cancer are listed contra-indications; the risks/benefits in individual cases should be considered carefully. Porphyria and active liver disease are absolute contraindications

Nutrition and blood

[9.1.1] Ferrous sulphate (OTC)

Tablets: 200 mg

Dose: adults only: usual dose 200 mg three times a day
                reduce dose if side effects occur

Side effects: nausea, epigastric pain, constipation (particularly in
                the elderly) or diarrhoea

Interactions: reduced absorption of iron with magnesium
                trisilicate, tetracyclines, biphosphonates, zinc

                iron reduces absorption of tetracyclines (e.g.
                doxycycline), quinolone antibiotics including
                ciprofloxacin, L-dopa and penicillamine

Caution: dangerous to children in overdose

[9.2.1.2] Dioralyte® (OTC)

Sachets: (blackcurrant, apricot, raspberry or plain) 20 per box,
                mix with 200 ml freshly boiled and cooled water, use
                within 1 h or keep in fridge.
                Sip frequently

Action: oral rehydration

Indication: fluid and electrolyte loss caused by diarrhoea, usually
                in infancy

Musculoskeletal system

[10.1.1] Ibuprofen (OTC)

Tablets:	200 mg (OTC), 400 mg (OTC), 600 mg
Suspension:	100 mg/5 ml

Dose:	all three times a day, ideally with food or milk
	adults: 400–600 mg
	children: under 1 year, or under 7 kg,
	              not recommended
	              1–2 years 2.5 ml
	              3–7 years 5 ml
	              8–12 years 10 ml

Side effects:	gastrointestinal discomfort – also nausea, diarrhoea, and occasionally bleeding and ulceration, hypersensitivity reactions – notably with bronchospasm, rashes and angioedema. Other rare side effects include fluid retention, headache, dizziness, vertigo, hearing disturbances such as tinnitus, photosensitivity, haematuria, blood disorders, renal failure, alveolitis, hepatic damage, pancreatitis, eye changes and aseptic meningitis
Cautions:	• gastrointestinal disease (especially peptic ulcer) • asthma (a small proportion of asthmatic patients find that ibuprofen worsens their symptoms; occasionally this can be severe) • allergy to aspirin or other NSAID • elderly, pregnancy, heart, kidney or liver disease • SLE

[10.3.2] Intralgin® (OTC)

Gel:	50 g pack
Dose:	apply liberally, massaging lightly three times a day
Side effect:	local irritation

Eye

[11.3.1] Chloramphenicol eye drops and ointment

Drops: 0.5%, 10 ml

Ointment: 1%, 4 g

Dose: drops   apply hourly at first
                        reduce to 4-hourly as symptoms improve
              ointment apply four times a day
                        or at night if used in conjunction with drops

Side effect: transient stinging

Cautions: history of aplastic anaemia
              discard 1 month after opening

[11.4.2] Sodium cromoglicate eye drops (OTC)

Eye drops: 2%, 13.5 ml

Dose: adults and children: 1 drop four times a day

Side effect: transient stinging

Caution: discard 1 month after opening

[11.8.1] Hypromellose eye drops (OTC)

Eye drops: 0.3%, 10 ml

Dose: apply as needed, usually 2 drops three times a day

Caution: discard 1 month after opening

Ear, nose and oropharynx

[12.1.1] Otosporin®

Ear drops:	5 ml, 10 ml contains two antibacterial agents: polymyxin B and neomycin; and one corticosteroid: hydrocortisone 1%
Dose:	2 drops three times a day
Side effect:	occasional local sensitivity reactions
Cautions:	avoid prolonged use if previous perforation, consult GP

[12.2.1] Beclometasone aqueous nasal spray (OTC)

Nasal spray:	beclometasone 50 µg per spray
Dose:	adults: two sprays to each nostril twice daily children over 6 years: as for adults
Side effects:	dry nose or throat, epistaxis, altered taste; rarely ulceration of the nasal septum, bronchospasm, raised intra-ocular pressure
Cautions:	untreated nasal infection, pulmonary tuberculosis in children, monitor height annually

[12.2.2] Saline nose drops (OTC)

Drops:	sodium chloride 0.9%, 10 ml
Dose:	apply to nostrils three times a day before feeds

[12.2.2] Warm moist air inhalation

Liquid: very hot water

Dose: inhale three or four times a day with a towel over the
                head

[12.3.1] Adcortyl in Orabase® (OTC)

Oral paste: 10 g

Dose: apply a thin layer two to four times daily, without
                rubbing in

Cautions: avoid using if there is oral infection (such as *herpes
                simplex*), history of peptic ulcer, diabetes, pregnancy

Skin

[13.2.1] **Emulsifying ointment 100 g/500 g; Hydrous ointment 100 g/500 g; Oilatum® 250 ml/500 ml; Sudocrem® 30 g/60 g/125 g/250 g/400 g** (all available OTC)

Dose: apply as frequently as necessary

Side effect: they can make the surface of a bath slippery

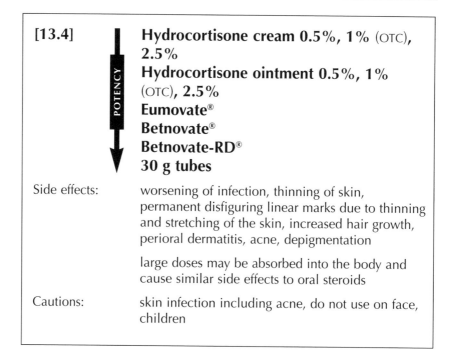

[13.4]   **Hydrocortisone cream 0.5%, 1%** (OTC), **2.5%**
                  Hydrocortisone ointment 0.5%, 1% (OTC), **2.5%**
                  Eumovate®
                  Betnovate®
                  Betnovate-RD®
                  30 g tubes

Side effects: worsening of infection, thinning of skin, permanent disfiguring linear marks due to thinning and stretching of the skin, increased hair growth, perioral dermatitis, acne, depigmentation

                 large doses may be absorbed into the body and cause similar side effects to oral steroids

Cautions: skin infection including acne, do not use on face, children

---

[13.4] **Miconazole/Hydrocortisone cream/ointment®**

Cream/ointment: 30 g containing miconazole 2% and hydrocortisone 1%

Dose: apply sparingly three times a day

Side effects: *see* hydrocortisone

Cautions: *see* hydrocortisone

[13.7] Glutaraldehyde (OTC)

Bottle: 10%, 10 ml

Administration: apply twice daily after soaking in warm soapy water for 3 minutes. Remove dead skin using an emery board

Side effect: local brown staining of skin

Cautions: do not apply to face or anogenital area, avoid healthy skin

[13.10.1] Fusidic acid

Cream or gel: 2%, 15, 30 g

Dose: apply three to four times a day

Side effect: rarely local hypersensitivity reactions

[13.10.3] Aciclovir cream (OTC)

Cream: 2 g (OTC), 10 g

Dose: apply every 4 h (five times a day) for 5 days at the first sign of an attack

Side effects: transient stinging or burning; occasionally erythema or drying of the skin

Interactions: interactions listed in the *BNF* apply to tablets and infusions, not this cream

Cautions: pregnancy – limited experience so best avoided avoid contact with mucous membranes

[13.10.4] Malathion (OTC)

Aqueous liquid 0.5% in bottles of 50 ml or 200 ml (100 ml per adult)

Administration and indications:

Head lice:	rub lotion into dry hair, comb, allow to dry wash off after 12 h repeat after 7 days
Scabies:	apply over whole body, excluding head and neck in adults do not wash hands after treatment wash off after 24 h
Side effect:	skin irritation
Cautions:	avoid contact with eyes, broken or infected skin

[13.10.4] Lyclear® (OTC)

Cream rinse 1%:	59 ml
Administration:	apply to clean damp hair, rinse off after 10 minutes and dry
Side effects:	itching, redness, stinging; rarely rashes, oedema
Cautions:	avoid contact with eyes, broken or infected skin pregnancy, breastfeeding, children under 6 months

Recommended reading

For the nurse

Edwards C and Stillman E (2000) *Minor Illness or Major Disease?* Pharmaceutical Press, London.

Fry J and Sandler G (1993) *Common Diseases: their nature, incidence and care.* Petroc Press, Newbury.

Guillebaud J (1998) *Contraception Today.* Martin Dunitz, London.

Neal M (1997) *Medical Pharmacology at a Glance.* Blackwell Science, Oxford.

Trounce J and Gould D (1999) *Clinical Pharmacology for Nurses.* Churchill Livingstone, London.

For the patient

Harvey S and Wylie I (1999) *Patient Power: getting the best from your healthcare.* Simon & Schuster, London.

McKenna P (1996) *Sleep Like a Log* (DVD and video). Sony Music.

Skynner R and Cleese J (1993) *Families and How to Survive Them.* Hutchinson Children's Books, London.

Trickett S (1990) *Sleep Like a Dream the Drug-free Way* (audiocassette). Potentials Unlimited.

Trickett S (1992) *Coping Successfully with Panic Attacks.* Sheldon Press, London.

Weekes C (2000) *Self-help for Your Nerves.* Thorsons, London.

Essential reference books

ABPI Compendium of Data Sheets and Summaries of Product Characteristics – published annually by Datapharm Publications.

British National Formulary (BNF) – updated every 6 months and published by the BMA and Royal Pharmaceutical Society of Great Britain.

Department of Health (1995) *Health Information for Overseas Travel*. The Stationery Office, London.

Department of Health (1996) *Immunisation Against Infectious Disease*. The Stationery Office, London.

OTC Directory – published annually by the Proprietary Society of Great Britain.

Ideas page

In our experience in managing minor illness, and from talking to doctors and nurses in other practices, we have encountered several treatments that appear both logical and effective. In the course of researching this book we have sought in vain for any evidence to support these treatments. We list them here to highlight the need for more evidence in these areas, and to invite readers' comments on their own experience of using them.

Boils

- the use of magnesium sulphate paste to 'draw' the purulent material from a boil

Ingrowing toenails

- teaching the patient to flick the corner of the nail away from the flesh daily

Pruritus

- sodium bicarbonate added to the bath (recommended in the NHS Direct Healthcare Guide)
- 2% menthol in aqueous cream
- witch hazel (for insect bites)

Haemorrhoids

- rectal cones (prescribable on FP10) for daily dilation of the anal canal until the condition resolves

Balanitis

- antibiotics such as fusidic acid in eye-drop form, to penetrate underneath the foreskin without leaving a sticky residue

Please contact us if you:

- have personal experience of using these treatments
- know of any good research in these areas
- would like to suggest other unproven treatments
- disagree with any of our recommendations, and have evidence to support your view.

Contact options:

Post: Stopsley Group Practice
             Wigmore Lane Health Centre
             Luton, Beds LU2 8BG

Website: www.minorillness.co.uk
E-mail: manual@minorillness.co.uk
Fax: 01582 456259

Glossary of medical abbreviations

bd/bid	twice daily
BMA	British Medical Association
BNF	*British National Formulary*
CXR	chest X-ray
△	diagnosis
EDD	expected date of delivery
ESR	erythrocyte sedimentation rate
FH	family history
FBC	full blood count
FP10	Prescription form (GP10 in Scotland)
FSH	Follicle-stimulating hormone
G6PD	glucose-6-phosphate dehydrogenase
GMS4	General Medical Services form
GP	general practitioner
HRT	hormone replacement therapy
HVS	high vaginal swab
i.m.	intramuscular
i.v.	intravenous
IUCD	intrauterine contraceptive device
LMP	last menstrual period
MAOI	monoamine oxidase inhibitor (class of anti-depressant drug)
MED 5	medical certificate used when the patient has not been seen by the signatory at the time of issue (pink)
MSU	mid-stream urine
NSAID	non-steroidal anti-inflammatory drug (e.g. ibuprofen)
od	once daily
OTC	over the counter (available without prescription)

PC4	post-coital contraceptive four-pill pack (contains oestrogen, unlike the levonorgestrel type)
PFR	peak flow rate
PMH	past medical history
prn	as required
p.v.	per vaginam (or indicating vaginal examination)
qds/qid	four times daily
RTA	road traffic accident
Rx	prescription or treatment
SC1	Self Certificate for time off work form 1
SC2	Self Certificate for time off work form 2
SLE	systemic lupus erythematosus
SSRI	selective serotonin re-uptake inhibitor (a type of anti-depressant)
tds/tid	three times daily
TFT	thyroid function test
UTI	urinary tract infection

Index